THE COMPLETE BOOK OF
NUTRITIONAL HEALING

THE COMPLETE BOOK
OF NUTRITIONAL HEALING
The Top 100 Medicinal Foods and Supplements
and the Diseases They Treat

Deborah Mitchell

Foreword by Hunter Yost, M.D.

A Lynn Sonberg Book

St. Martin's Paperbacks

Notice: This book is intended as a reference volume only, not as a medical manual. The information given here is designed to help you make informed decisions about your health. It is not intended as a substitute for any treatment that may have been prescribed by your doctor. If you suspect that you have a medical problem, we urge you to seek competent medical help.

Mention of specific companies, organizations, or authorities in this book does not imply endorsement by the author or publisher, nor does mention of specific companies, organizations, or authorities imply that they endorse this book, its author or the publisher.

Internet addresses given in this book were accurate at the time it went to press.

THE COMPLETE BOOK OF NUTRITIONAL HEALING

Copyright © 2008 by Lynn Sonberg Book Associates.

Cover photo © Brian Hagiwara/FoodPix.

All rights reserved.

For information address St. Martin's Press, 175 Fifth Avenue, New York, NY 10010.

ISBN: 0-312-94511-6
EAN: 978-0-312-94511-4

Printed in the United States of America

St. Martin's Paperbacks edition / January 2009

St. Martin's Paperbacks are published by St. Martin's Press, 175 Fifth Avenue, New York, NY 10010.

10 9 8 7 6 5 4 3

CONTENTS

PART II: MEDICINAL FOODS AND SUPPLEMENTS
Top 80+ Medicinal Foods

Top 20 Supplements

FOREWORD

This practical and up-to-date handbook provides the perfect natural and nutritional antidotes for the chronic ills of the Western diet and lifestyle. The medical literature over the past several years clearly recommends nutritional and lifestyle changes as the first line of therapy for most of the major chronic diseases, including heart disease, high blood pressure, diabetes, obesity, osteoporosis, arthritis and metabolic syndrome, instead of drugs.[1] These and many other chronic diseases are imminently preventable, yet account for seventy-eight percent of all health care expenses in the U.S.[2] Other studies indicate that doctors do not spend time discussing nutritional therapies with their patients.[3]

The vegetables and fruits listed in this book contain a treasure trove of complex phytonutrients that are proven to positively influence genetic expression to prevent cancer and many chronic diseases in ways no pharmaceutical drug ever could. Genes are not destiny and good nutrition can make a huge difference. Emphasizing plant-based proteins over animal-based proteins sends positive chemical signals to decrease inflammation all over the body, protecting blood vessels, joints and organs. Many common prescription medications can deplete essential nutrients, leading to more health problems. The supplements in this book will help complete a well-rounded nutritional program. Described herein are the keys to good health and longevity, the low-technology approaches of healthy nutrition and lifestyle.

Rather than wait years for the information contained in this book to be incorporated into the daily practice habits of the average primary-care physician, readers can begin today to use these safe, simple and well-researched suggestions to improve their health. This book fulfills Franklin's dictum quite well: "An ounce of prevention is worth a pound of cure."

Hunter Yost, M.D. (www.hunteryostmd.com)

1. Roberts, CK. Bernard, RJ. Effects of diet and exercise on chronic disease. J App Physiol 2005; 98 (1):3–30.
2. Holman, H. Chronic Disease—The need for a new clinical education. JAMA 2004; 292(9):1057–1059.
3. Ashley, JM et. al. Weight control in the physician's office. Arch. Intern Med 2001; 161:1599–1604.

INTRODUCTION

"To eat is a necessity, but to eat intelligently is an art."
—*La Rochefaucauld*

Welcome to this handy, comprehensive guide to intelligent, fun, and healthy eating. For your convenience, we have gathered together the latest information on food, supplements, and health challenges, and presented it in a way that allows you to browse, think about what you've read, savor it (yes, we've included some easy-to-follow recipes), check references if you are curious, and use what you've learned to enhance your health and that of your family.

How do we do that? First we look at what's ailing you; and then we introduce foods and supplements that will allow you to improve your health and that of your family by eating intelligently. Eating smart can be enjoyable and it definitely can be delicious, but it also has a serious side: according to the US Department of Health and Human Services, an unhealthy diet and inactivity cause 310,000 to 580,000 deaths in the United States every year. By making wise food choices, with the help of this book, you can better ensure you and your family will never be a part of this statistic.

FIFTY-PLUS HEALTH CHALLENGES

"The doctor of the future will give no medicine, but will interest his patients in the care of the human frame, diet and in the
cause and prevention of diseases."

— *Thomas A. Edison*

It's safe to say that no one gets through life without experiencing at least a few minor health challenges. Most young children get ear infections, the vast majority of teenagers have a
bout of acne, and do you know anyone who hasn't ever had a
cold or a headache? Heart disease is the number one killer of
women in the United States, more than fifty percent of adults
are overweight, more than forty million Americans either
have diabetes or are at high risk for the disease, and all women
can look forward to menopause.

These are just a few of the common health and medical conditions discussed in the first part of this book. These conditions
were selected based on two main criteria: (1) they are common
ailments or diseases that affect a great number of people regardless of age, although the vast majority of the conditions
chosen occur mostly in adults; and (2) there are foods and/or
supplements that may help prevent, treat, and/or manage these
conditions, based largely on scientific research and study results from a wide variety of sources.

Each health challenge entry addresses three issues: background information, causes, and how foods and supplements
may help. If you turn to the entry for "Gingivitis," for example, you will learn how you could help prevent and treat this
common dental disease with the supplement coenzyme Q10
(CoQ10), foods rich in vitamin C (for healthy gums), cranberries (help prevent bacteria from sticking to your teeth), and
green tea (contains catechins that fight plaque). You can then
turn to Part II where there are individual detailed entries for
each of the foods and supplements suggested.

HEALING FOODS

"The art of medicine consists of amusing the patient while nature cures the disease."

—*Voltaire*

Some of the best cures and disease-fighting options come in the form of delicious foods that also provide a dazzling variety of nutrients. When you break through the peel of an orange, bite into a crisp almond, or savor the warm goodness of a bowl of oatmeal, you are getting more than great taste—you are getting a dose of Nature's medicine.

Nature has some very inventive ways of packaging her many healing elements—in berries and leaves, fruits and stems, roots and rhizomes. Sometimes her offerings come from the animal kingdom. The eighty-plus foods chosen for this book were selected because they offer good to excellent amounts of various nutrients that have been shown scientifically to benefit human health. Research has suggested that they may help reduce the risk of some of our more serious medical challenges—cancer, diabetes, heart disease, stroke, obesity, among others. Most of the chosen foods are also nutrient dense, which means the amount of nutrients a food contains is high when compared with the number of calories it provides. To optimize the nutritional value of the foods discussed, we encourage you to buy organic foods whenever possible.

Why "eighty-plus"? A few of the entries discuss more than one food item under a broader category. For example, "Beans" provides information on black, kidney, and pinto beans, among others. Beans is a food category that has many members with enough nutritional similarities to warrant discussing them in one entry, but a few differences that are worth highlighting separately.

The foods explored in this section are all familiar ones—you won't need to go to an exotic natural food market to find them—and they are mainly whole foods, or, in a few cases, foods that have undergone minimal processing. And they taste great. If you don't believe us, let the proof be in the tasting! To help you along, we provide two recipes in each food entry (or in a few cases, tips on how to use the food) so you can discover on your own just how good these foods are and how easily you can include them in your daily diet.

Overall, each entry in the healing foods section is brimming with concise, relevant information that we have broken down as follows:

- background information on the food
- nutritional data (see detailed discussion below)
- health benefits of each food item, with an emphasis on the ailments discussed in "Fifty-Plus Health Challenges" and the supplements covered in "Nutritional Supplements"
- how to select and store the item, with tips on how to get the most nutritional value from the food
- recipes and/or tips on how to use the item

Nutritional Information

To help you better understand the nutritional value of each of the foods we discuss, the "Nutrition" heading in each entry lists the amount of calories, total fat, protein, carbohydrates, fiber, and cholesterol, as well as the amount of selected nutrients and their "DRI" values. The "DRI" is Dietary Reference Intake, which is an updated and expanded version of the RDA, or Recommended Daily Allowance. In 1997, the Food and Nutrition Board of the National Academy of Sciences began the process of revising the RDAs.

Part of the revision process involved creating DRIs, which take into account not only the amount of a nutrient needed to prevent a deficiency (which is what the RDA was based upon), but to also consider what it would take to reduce the risk of chronic diseases, such as heart disease, diabetes, cancer, and liver and kidney disease. For some nutrients, the DRI values are the same for both sexes. The DRI for folic acid, for example, is 400 mcg for both men and women. If a food contains 40 mcg of folic acid per serving, we present the information as: "Folic acid: 40 mcg, 10% DRI." In other cases the established values for men and women are different. In those instances, we have used an average of the two values as the standard. For example, the DRI for vitamin K is 120 mcg for men and 90 mcg for women, so we have used 105 mcg as the standard.

Phytonutrients

In addition to the nutrients listed for each food entry, many of which are items you can see on a "Nutrition Facts" label on foods in the supermarket, most healing foods also contain other important nutrients called phytochemicals or phytonutrients ("phyto" means "plant"). Phytonutrients are non-vitamin, non-mineral organic components found in plants that appear to provide three major purposes in the human body: they act as antioxidants (preventing development of or destroying free radicals) associated with diseases and aging, they regulate hormone levels, and they eliminate toxins.

We talk about phytonutrients throughout this book, so you may want to familiarize yourself with a few of the more common classes and how they can benefit you.

- Carotenoids: These are plant pigments, which give plants their colors. Some common carotenoids include alpha-carotene, beta-carotene, lutein, lycopene, and zeaxanthin. They act as antioxidants and also enhance the immune system, facilitate cell-to-cell communications, and protect the skin against ultraviolet radiation.
- Flavonoids: This category includes anthocyanins, catechins, ellagic acid, flavonols, isoflavones, quercetin, and resveratrol. These antioxidants also prevent blood clotting, protect against heart disease, lower harmful estrogen levels, protect the eyes, and improve symptoms of allergy and arthritis.
- Indoles and isothiocyanates: These are found mainly in cruciferous vegetables (e.g., broccoli, cauliflower, kale) and help reduce cancer risk by activating enzymes that detoxify carcinogens, lower levels of harmful estrogen, and suppress tumor growth.
- Lignans: These substances are insoluble fibers that act

as antioxidants. They are found mainly in whole grains and berries.

- Phenols: Found in nearly all fruits, vegetables, and grains, they act as antioxidants, prevent blood clots, activate enzymes that fight cancer, and prevent inflammation.
- Phytates: These phosphorus compounds are found mainly in cereal grains, nuts, and legumes. They may help prevent the formation of free radicals.
- Saponins: Tomatoes, garlic, onions, and spinach host these phytonutrients, which help block the absorption of cholesterol and lower the amount of fats circulating in the bloodstream.
- Sulfides: Also known as organosulfurs, they are found in chives, garlic, leeks, onions, and shallots. They fight bacterial, fungal, and viral infections, reduce blood glucose levels, enhance circulation, and may help prevent heart disease by lowering cholesterol.

How do phytonutrients differ from vitamins and minerals? The most obvious difference is that they come from plants, but another difference is that there are thousands of different types of phytonutrients, compared with a few dozen vitamins and minerals. Each phytonutrient has distinct functions and characteristics, many of which may be still unknown. That's because phytonutrients are a relatively new discovery, and so the body of knowledge and research is very limited, especially compared with what we know about vitamins and minerals.

Because experts do know more about vitamins and minerals, they have been able to establish DRIs for most of them. This feature has not been applied to phytonutrients. However, as experts learn more about phytonutrients, DRIs for individual nutrients may be available in the near future.

NUTRITIONAL SUPPLEMENTS

Next we introduce twenty important nutrients that are available in supplement form as well as in foods, especially those discussed in the "Healing Foods" section. Each entry in this section provides the following:

- background information on the nutrient
- health benefits associated with its use, focusing on ailments discussed in "Fifty-Plus Health Challenges" that may benefit from the nutrient
- how much you need to use
- possible interactions with drugs and/or other nutrients when using this supplement
- food sources of the nutrient, with a focus on those discussed in the "Healing Foods" section

This section is helpful in two ways. One, you can learn about specific supplements that you may be taking or may be considering to see if they are a good fit for your health needs and lifestyle. Two, you can quickly see which healing foods are good sources of these nutrients.

Finally, we want to say that the information for this book was gathered from a wide range of print and electronic sources, including the American Dietetic Association, American Heart Association, Center for Science in the Public Interest, Cleveland Clinic, Food and Drug Administration, Mayo Clinic, and the US Department of Agriculture National Nutrient Data Laboratory, among others, as well as the research results from articles in dozens of medical journals. If you want to learn more about any of the foods, supplements, or health conditions covered in this book, see the detailed, alphabetized note section at the end of the book, where you can find sources for the information presented in each entry.

The choice is up to you: starting right now you can eat smarter and healthier. You can feel good about the food you give yourself and your family, knowing that it not only tastes great but that it has the potential to enhance your life with every bite. Just turn the page and begin.

PART I
Fifty-Plus Health Challenges

ACNE

Acne (*acne vulgaris*) is a chronic inflammatory skin condition characterized by lesions that typically appear on the face and neck, but also on the back, chest, shoulders, and upper arms. Eighty to ninety-five percent of adolescents develop acne.

To diagnose acne, doctors usually just need to examine the skin. Typical symptoms include redness and/or skin inflammation, and the formation of lesions—e.g., whiteheads, blackheads, cysts, and/or abscesses. Symptoms can range from mild to severe.

What Causes Acne?

Experts generally agree that what you eat does not cause acne; rather, they point to family history, hormone imbalances (typical of adolescence), stress, and a weakened immune system. However, studies show that the Western diet in general (which is high in fat, sugar, and refined carbohydrates) can promote acne. In some cases, acne is caused by medications, such as corticosteroids or phenytoin; or by an endocrine disorder, including Cushing's disease or polycystic ovary syndrome.

Skin eruptions occur when the pores in the skin are blocked. This blockage happens during adolescence, when an increase in hormone levels raises production of sebum, a substance that lubricates the skin, and keratin, a component of hair. These two substances can clog hair follicles, causing whiteheads and blackheads to form. If the trapped bacteria interact with the oil, inflammation can occur and more severe lesions may develop.

Acne usually disappears after adolescence, although it does affect about twelve percent of women (especially those in perimenopause) and three percent of men. Most lesions don't leave lasting scars unless you pick at them.

How Foods and Supplements Can Help

A "clean" diet—fresh, organic fruits and vegetables (see individual fruits and vegetables in Part II), reduced intake of saturated fat and processed sugar, drinking filtered water, eating only hormone-free dairy products—can help minimize symptoms. Supplements may also help: vitamin A (as beta-carotene, 5,000 IU daily) and vitamin E (400 IU daily) can reduce inflammation, as can zinc (30 mg zinc gluconate) and omega-3 fatty acids (1,000 mg daily). Zinc also kills Propionibacterium acnes, the main bacteria associated with acne. If you have acne associated with perimenopause, take 25 to 50 mg of vitamin B-6 two to three times per day.

Foods rich in vitamin A (sweet potatoes, carrots, greens), vitamin E (olive oil, avocados, greens), zinc (wheat germ, pumpkin seeds), and omega-3s (salmon, tuna) are also beneficial.

ALLERGIES/ASTHMA

An allergy is any negative or abnormal reaction by the immune system to a substance (an allergen) that is usually harmless but which the body interprets as a threat. An estimated twenty percent of people have allergies. Asthma is a chronic respiratory condition in which the airways in the lungs become swollen. When airways are inflamed, they are very sensitive and respond to various substances to which people are allergic, which can make it difficult to breathe.

What Causes Allergies?

Whether the offending allergen is pollen, the venom from a bee sting, or an antibiotic, the immune system reacts in a similar way: the body produces a specific antibody, called IgE, which attaches to the allergens, which in turn bind to special blood cells called mast cells. This process triggers the release of various chemicals, including histamine, which causes most of the symptoms associated with allergies. For example, a respiratory allergy, such as hayfever, typically causes sneezing, itchy eyes, and nasal congestion, while a food allergy can cause vomiting, stomach pain, and diarrhea, and a drug allergy may produce rash, breathing difficulties, and swelling. Symptoms are usually mild to moderate, but in rare cases a severe, life-threatening reaction called anaphylaxis occurs.

Children can inherit the tendency to be allergic from their parents, but they do not inherit an allergy to a specific allergen. To identify allergens, allergists can use skin testing, which is the most common and effective approach; blood tests; and an elimination technique in which people remove certain allergens from their life and then reintroduce them to see if they react.

What Causes Asthma?

Asthma can be caused by many different factors, including allergens (e.g., pollen, dust, pet dander), irritants (e.g., air pollution, chemicals, cigarette smoke), or other substances, as well as circumstances (e.g., exercise, emotional stress). Symptoms include wheezing, tight chest, difficulty breathing, and cough.

About twenty million people have asthma in the United States, and nearly half of them are children. Most people who have asthma also have allergies, and children with a family history of allergies and asthma are more likely to have the disease. To establish a diagnosis of asthma, doctors may use allergy testing, X-rays, or a spirometer, which measures how much air is exhaled after taking a deep breath.

How Foods and Supplements Can Help

Foods rich in vitamin E and vitamin E supplements can help reduce the severity of hayfever symptoms, so be sure to enjoy almonds, walnuts, pumpkin seeds, greens, and eggs. Vitamin C is a natural antihistamine, and taking 10 to 30 mg daily for every two pounds of body weight can be beneficial.

Coenzyme Q10 is an antihistamine as well; 50 to 150 mg daily is recommended.

People with asthma often respond well to omega-3 fatty acids, both as a supplement (1,000 mg daily) and as part of their diet. In fact, studies recommend eating omega-3–rich fish, such as salmon and tuna, three times a week. Magnesium supplements (250–500 mg daily) along with magnesium-rich foods (almonds, avocado, beans [dried], greens, peas, pumpkin seeds, tofu) may relieve breathing difficulties in people with asthma, while research also indicates that antioxidants, including vitamins C and E, found in fruits and vegetables help reduce asthma symptoms.

ANEMIA

Anemia is a blood disease in which there is a deficiency of red blood cells or hemoglobin, a substance in the blood that contains iron. In people who have anemia, the hemoglobin in their blood does not transport enough oxygen to the rest of the body. When the body doesn't get the oxygen it needs, fatigue and weakness result.

About twenty percent of women and three percent of men have anemia. Anemia can be temporary or long-term, with mild to severe symptoms, and it can be diagnosed using a routine blood test.

What Causes Anemia?

Although anemia can be caused by several factors, the most common cause is an insufficient amount of iron. The body needs iron to make hemoglobin: thus a deficiency of iron equals a deficiency of hemoglobin, which results in anemia. Low iron levels can be caused by pregnancy, an iron-poor diet, or blood loss due to colon cancer, ulcers, colon polyps, or heavy menstrual flow.

Other causes of anemia include a vitamin deficiency (folate and/or vitamin B-12), sickle cell anemia, Crohn's disease, rheumatoid arthritis, chemotherapy, bone or blood cancers, an intestinal disorder that affects the absorption of nutrients, and kidney disease. Along with fatigue and weakness, people with anemia often feel sluggish, dizzy, cold, and irritable. Headache, rapid or irregular heartbeat, and pale skin are also common.

How Foods and Supplements Can Help

Before you treat anemia with iron supplements and/or iron-rich foods, you should undergo blood testing to make sure you are iron deficient, as iron is toxic if taken in large amounts. Iron-rich foods include beans, lentils, iron-fortified cereals, fortified oatmeal, tofu, and leafy greens. For an iron supplement, a recommended dose is 30 mg of succinate, gluconate, or fumarate iron, twice daily between meals. If you experience stomach discomfort, take 30 mg with meals three times daily. Because vitamin C assists in iron absorption, take 1,000 mg three times daily with meals.

If you have a vitamin B-12 anemia, you can take sublingual supplements of the vitamin (2,000 mcg three times daily for 30 days). After 30 days, take 1,000 mcg methylcobalamin (a form of B-12) once daily. Foods rich in vitamin B-12 should be a part of your diet as well, and include salmon, fortified cereals, yogurt, and tuna. For anemia associated with a folic acid deficiency, or to support treatment of an iron or B-12–associated anemia, take 800 mcg folic acid three times daily. Foods rich in folic acid include asparagus, avocados, bananas, beans, beets, celery, greens, oranges, and peas.

Nutrients that support production of red blood cells include vitamin B-5 (take 25 to 100 mg daily) and vitamin B-6 (take 25 to 100 mg daily). Foods rich in vitamin B-5 include wheat bran, peas, broccoli, mushrooms, and sweet potatoes; for vitamin B-6, consider almonds, avocados, bananas, beans, brown rice, lentils, turkey, salmon, and walnuts.

ARTHRITIS

Arthritis is a general term that describes a condition in which people experience inflammation or pain in one or more joints.

The most common form of arthritis is osteoarthritis, a degenerative disease that affects more than forty million people in the United States. Osteoarthritis usually affects people who are sixty-five years or older, and causes joint stiffness when rising in the morning and painful joints that worsen with movement.

Rheumatoid arthritis is an autoimmune disease, which means the body mistakenly recognizes parts of the body as being foreign and attacks them. If you have rheumatoid arthritis, the attack results in inflammation in the joints and, in some cases, the surrounding tissues (e.g., muscles, tendons, ligaments) and organs as well. About two million Americans have rheumatoid arthritis, and it generally first appears between the ages of forty and sixty.

What Causes Arthritis?

Osteoarthritis is caused by wear and tear on the joints, which in turn places stress on the structures that support the cartilage. Once the cartilage is damaged, enzymes are released that destroy the cartilage in the joints. Joints in the hands, feet, spine, hips, and knees are most affected. The pain is caused by the joint ends rubbing together and the thinning of the cartilage.

Experts are not certain what causes rheumatoid arthritis. Some believe heredity is involved; others say an infection or environmental factors cause the body to attack itself. Regardless of what triggers the disease, the immune system responds by activating cells called lymphocytes and sending special chemicals to the joints. The inflammation in the joints causes pain, redness, swelling, and stiffness. Fatigue, low fever, muscle aches, and lack of appetite are also common.

How Foods and Supplements Can Help

To help prevent bone loss, supplementation with calcium (1,000 mg daily) along with magnesium (500 mg daily) and foods rich in calcium (e.g., almonds, brewer's yeast, broccoli, greens, nonfat milk, seaweed, tofu, yogurt) are recommended. Folate and B-6 are important, as studies show that inflammation quickly destroys these B vitamins in people who have rheumatoid arthritis. Supplements of folate (400 mcg twice daily) and B-6 (25–100 mg daily) are suggested, along with good food sources: avocados, bananas, beans, beets, brown rice, celery, greens, lentils, oranges, and walnuts, for example.

Research also shows that omega-3 can relieve tender joints and decrease morning stiffness in people who have rheumatoid arthritis, and that diets rich in omega-3 and low in omega-6 fatty acids (found in high levels in most vegetable oils and in lower amounts in meat) can benefit people who have osteoarthritis. An omega-3 supplement (3–5 g daily, containing EPA and DHA) can be helpful, as can eating flaxseed, herring, salmon, sardines, tuna, and walnuts.

A diet that includes many fruits and vegetables, which are excellent sources of antioxidants (e.g., vitamins C and E, beta-carotene, and selenium) is recommended for arthritis. In fact, studies show that the risk of rheumatoid arthritis is highest among people who consume the lowest amounts of antioxidants. Some foods that are rich in antioxidants are berries (e.g., blueberries, cranberries, strawberries) and yellow and green vegetables (e.g., squashes, sweet potatoes, carrots, cabbage). Also, a plant-based diet can be very beneficial for people with rheumatoid arthritis, because it eliminates arachidonic acid, which is found in meat products and causes inflammation.

ATHEROSCLEROSIS

Atherosclerosis is a type of arteriosclerosis, which is a general term for the thickening and hardening of arteries. Atherosclerosis comes from the Greek "athero" (meaning paste) and "sclerosis (hardness) and is the process by which deposits of cholesterol, calcium, and other substances accumulate in the inner lining of the arteries. This buildup, called plaque, can eventually block the flow of blood through an artery and/or rupture and cause blood clots to form. These clots can impair blood flow anywhere in the body, including the brain, heart, kidneys, arms, and legs. If blood flow to the heart is blocked, it causes a heart attack; if flow to the brain is hindered, a stroke results.

What Causes Atherosclerosis?

Atherosclerosis is a slowly progressing disease that starts when the innermost layer of the arteries is damaged by factors such as high levels of triglycerides and/or cholesterol, high blood pressure, tobacco smoke, or diabetes. Much of this damage often begins in childhood and is related to diet: high-fat, fried, and sugary foods, combined with a lack of adequate exercise, contribute to atherosclerosis. With age, the combination of diet and other factors results in hardening of the arteries.

Symptoms of atherosclerosis do not usually appear until about forty percent of an artery is blocked, and symptoms vary depending on which vessels are affected. When an artery that provides oxygen-rich blood to the heart is partly blocked, chest pain (angina) can occur; if an artery is completely blocked, a heart attack may result. Blockage of an artery leading to the brain can cause a stroke, while impeded blood flow to an extremity can cause significant pain, numbness, loss of mobility, and gangrene.

How Foods and Supplements Can Help

Since diet is a major factor in atherosclerosis, there is much you can do to prevent and treat this disease. Generally, choose a diet based on fresh fruits and vegetables, whole grains and legumes, with minimal low-fat dairy and animal protein. In addition, specific foods and supplements can be especially helpful.

Folic acid, for example, helps lower levels of homocysteine, a substance that contributes to atherosclerosis. Foods rich in folic acid include asparagus, avocado, beans (dried), lentils, and greens; you may also consider a supplement, 400–800 mcg daily. Folic acid should be accompanied by vitamin B-12, which can be found primarily in animal products (e.g., meat, poultry, fish); 100–300 mcg daily as a supplement is the suggested dose.

Since free-radical damage is a hallmark of atherosclerosis, antioxidants can be most helpful. Foods with high levels of vitamin C, vitamin E, beta-carotene, quercetin, and selenium are recommended, especially apples, artichokes, asparagus, avocados, barley, blueberries, broccoli, carrots, cantaloupe, cauliflower, garlic, grapes, mushrooms, onions, parsley, sea-weed, tea, tomatoes, turnips, and watermelon. Suggested supplement doses per day include: vitamin C, 100–1,000 mg; vitamin E, 100–800 IU; beta-carotene, 5,000 IU; quercetain, 35 mg; selenium, 200 mcg.

ATHLETE'S FOOT

You don't need to be an athlete to suffer the itching, burning, and inflammation associated with athlete's foot. Also known as *tinea pedis*, this annoying and uncomfortable superficial fungal infection typically affects the skin between the toes, but it can also attack the toenails, soles, and sides of the feet. It is mildly contagious, but it is also preventable and treatable.

What Causes Athlete's Foot?

Athlete's foot is caused by a fungus called dermatophytes that thrives in damp, warm, close environments like the inside of your shoes and socks, or in locker rooms and showers. The fungus can be transported on flaking skin from infected feet and be passed along to other people on shower floors, rugs, clothing, shoes, and other surfaces. Men are more likely than women to get athlete's foot; other people at risk include anyone who has a weakened immune system due to diabetes, HIV/AIDS, or other chronic disease, or anyone who takes an antibiotic for two weeks or longer.

To help prevent athlete's foot, keep your feet dry, especially between your toes. If your feet tend to sweat a lot, change your socks often, wear sandals or shoes that allow your feet to "breathe," and go barefoot when possible. When in fitness centers, communal showers, or similar places, wear waterproof shoes or sandals.

How Foods and Supplements Can Help

Athlete's foot is a condition in which some foods are helpful if they are eaten *and* applied to the feet. Take garlic for example. Garlic is an excellent antifungal, and including several cloves per day in your diet can help eliminate athlete's foot. However, you can also place slivers of fresh garlic in your socks or shoes for several hours a day to kill the fungus.

Cinnamon and ginger also have antifungal powers, and you can make a tea using one or both that you can drink *and* soak your feet in (two different batches, naturally; the foot soak decoction should be stronger than the tea). For a ginger treatment, for example, add one ounce of chopped ginger root to eight ounces of boiling water. Simmer for twenty minutes and apply the solution to the problem areas twice a day using a clean cloth or cotton ball. If you prefer cinnamon, boil two cups of water, add five broken cinnamon sticks, and simmer for five minutes. Remove from the heat and let it steep, covered, for forty-five minutes, before using as a foot soak.

Vitamin E, applied topically or taken as a supplement, can help eliminate athlete's foot. Take 300 to 400 IU daily as a supplement, or break open a capsule and apply the contents to the affected area twice a day until the infection has cleared. Zinc may also help: take 30 mg daily to boost the immune system. Good food sources of zinc include eggs, pumpkin seeds, wheat germ, and yogurt.

Speaking of yogurt, look for varieties that contain lots of probiotics—good bacteria that can help restore immune system health. As a supplement, take two to three billion units daily of a probiotics supplement that contains at least four different species of beneficial bacteria (e.g., Lactobacillus and Bifidobacterium species).

BRONCHITIS

Bronchitis is inflammation, infection, or irritation of the bronchi (breathing tubes) in the upper portion of the lungs. In many cases, bronchitis begins as a cough that develops after a bout of the common cold, flu, or other respiratory condition. Within a day or two of the cough's appearance, symptoms such as fever, chills, tightness of the chest, and phlegm production occur. Such cases of acute bronchitis typically disappear within a week or so, although the cough may linger. In some people, especially those who are overweight, sedentary, or who smoke, bronchitis may become chronic.

What Causes Bronchitis?

Acute bronchitis is usually caused by the same viruses that cause colds and flu, but a small percentage of people get the disease after being exposed to cigarette smoke, air pollutants or smog, or even from gastroesophageal reflux disease (GERD). The major cause of chronic bronchitis is smoking.

How Foods and Supplements Can Help

To prevent and treat bronchitis, it's important to boost and support your immune system and to detoxify your body.

- The antioxidants beta-carotene (take 5,000–15,000 IU daily) and vitamin C (3,000 mg daily in divided doses) can help protect the lungs. Good food sources of beta-carotene (e.g., carrots, greens, pumpkin, squash, sweet potatoes) and vitamin C (e.g., bell peppers, blueberries, cantaloupe, citrus, greens, mango, papaya, parsley, peaches, peas, tomatoes, watermelon) should also be included in your diet.
- The bioflavonoid quercetin, 1,000 mg daily in divided doses along with vitamin C, is also suggested. Red apples, red grapes, red onions, tea, and red wine are good food sources of quercetin.
- Zinc can help promote healing of the bronchial tubes and support the immune system. To treat an acute case of bronchitis, a suggested dose is 15 mg daily. Foods that provide a healthy amount of zinc include eggs, pumpkin seeds, wheat germ, and yogurt.

BURSITIS

Bursitis is inflammation of one or more of the 150-plus tiny fluid-filled sacs, called bursae, in the body. Bursae are located near your joints, such as the shoulders, knees, elbows, hips, and ankles, where they help reduce friction between bones, tendons, and ligaments throughout the body. When the bursae become inflamed, they can cause pain, limited immobility, and tenderness. Bursitis that does not involve an infection of the fluid can usually be treated without medication; if infection occurs, antibiotics may be necessary.

What Causes Bursitis?

The most common causes of bursitis are overuse, repetitive motion, and trauma to a joint. If you play tennis or golf, kneel while gardening, use a vacuum cleaner, or have a job that requires repetitive movements like working on an assembly line, then you may develop bursitis. Bursitis may also result from arthritis, an infection, or gout.

The most common form of bursitis is olecranon bursitis, in which a tender swelling appears just behind the elbow. Because the elbow is involved in a great deal of repeated motion and is susceptible to injury, healing can take a long time and infection is common.

How Foods and Supplements Can Help

The main goal when treating bursitis is to eliminate the inflammation. Omega-3 fatty acids, as a supplement (1,000 mg twice daily) and/or in foods such as flaxseed, salmon, tuna, and walnuts, can be helpful. To assist with healing of irritated tissue, supplementing with vitamin C (250–500 mg twice daily) along with foods rich in vitamin C (e.g., bell peppers, blueberries, cantaloupe, guava, kiwi, papaya, oranges) can be beneficial.

Consider going Hawaiian and include pineapple in your daily diet. Pineapple is rich in bromelain, a natural anti-inflammatory substance, which is also available as a supplement.

CANCER

Cancer is the uncontrolled reproduction and growth of cells that results in a tumor or similar abnormal growth. More than one hundred different types of cancer have been identified, and they fall into four main categories: carcinomas (those affecting the skin, mucous membranes, glands, and other organs); leukemias (blood cancers), lymphomas (in the lymphatic system); and sarcomas (found in bone, connective tissue, and muscle).

Although currently there are no cures for cancer, there is much you can do to prevent it, as well as treat the disease and improve quality of life.

What Causes Cancer?

All types of cancer are caused by a basic factor: there is a mutation in the nucleus of a cell, which can be triggered by any number of factors, and the result is the growth of abnormal cells. Some known or suspected carcinogens—substances that trigger or stimulate the mutation process—include cigarette smoke, sunlight, radiation, and chemicals found in pesticides, household cleaners, paints, food, clothing, water, air, and other everyday items.

How Foods and Supplements Can Help

Just as there are many different types of cancer, there are also many foods and nutrients that may help prevent cancer. Foods high in fiber, for example, can help prevent colon cancer, while foods rich in antioxidants may protect the body against cancer-triggering damage caused by free radicals. In fact, if a food is known to protect against one type of cancer, it usually is also beneficial against others as well. Therefore, the following is a list of foods that have anticancer properties. Those that have been shown to be especially helpful against a specific type of cancer are noted. However, include as many of these foods as possible: apricots, barley, beans (dried), beets, bell peppers, blueberries, broccoli, brown rice, bulgar, carrots, cantaloupe, cruciferous vegetables (e.g., Brussel sprouts, cabbage, cauliflower, radishes [prostate and colon cancer]), flaxseed, garlic, grapefruit, greens, guava, kefir, lentils, mangoes, oats, olive oil, onions, oranges, papaya, pomegranates (prostate cancer), quinoa, seaweed, soy, strawberries, tea (ovarian cancer, associated with the kaempferol found in tea), tomatoes, turmeric, turnips, watermelon, wheat germ, and yogurt.

Experts have also identified some individual supplements that have cancer-fighting properties. A report presented at the American Association for Cancer Research noted that an increased intake of vitamin D reduced the risk of breast cancer by fifty percent. In another study on breast cancer, researchers found that the risk of the disease was forty-six percent less among postmenopausal women who consumed the most flavonoids compared with those who consumed the least. And in a Harvard study, researchers found that vitamin D significantly improved survival rates among people with lung cancer. Doses of 1,100 IU were used in some studies; the upper tolerable limit for vitamin D is 2,000 IU daily.

On the spicy side, some experts credit curcumin (a component of turmeric) with cancer-protective effects. In a 2007 report, Bharat B. Aggarwal, PhD, of the University of Texas M. D. Anderson Cancer Center, noted that "Among all the cancers we and others have examined, no cancer yet has been found which is not affected by curcumin." A suggested dose is 400 to 600 mg of standardized curcumin powder three times daily.

CANKER SORES

Ouch! It can be painful to eat, drink, even talk, when you have canker sores. Unlike fever blisters, which develop on the outside of the mouth, canker sores (aphthous stomatitis) usually form on the inside of the lips or cheeks, at the base of the gums, or under the tongue. They appear as white or yellow spots surrounded by a bright red area. Up to eighty-five percent of the US population experiences at least one episode of canker sores during their lifetime. Women, adolescents, and twenty-somethings are those most likely to get canker sores, but they can develop in anyone. The good news is that they are not contagious and that they typically go away after a few weeks without treatment.

What Causes Canker Sores?

No definitive cause of canker sores has been identified, but many experts believe they may be triggered by poor nutrition (especially deficiencies of folic acid and/or vitamin B-12), food allergies, menstruation, aggressive teeth brushing, hormonal changes (as during adolescence), or emotional stress. People who occasionally or frequently bite their tongue or the inside of their cheeks often develop canker sores. The pain usually subsides over seven to ten days and the sores disappear within two to three weeks.

How Foods and Supplements Can Help

Although canker sores typically go away without treatment, you can speed up the healing process as well as help prevent future episodes by making a few wise food and supplement choices. Make sure you get enough folic acid (take 400 mcg daily as a supplement) and vitamin B-12 (400 mcg daily). Food choices for folic acid include asparagus, avocado, beans (dried), beets, bell peppers, broccoli, cabbage, cauliflower, corn, fortified cereals, greens, oranges, papaya, parsnips, peas, soybeans, tofu, turkey, wheat germ; for vitamin B-12, clams, fortified cereals, salmon, tuna, turkey.

Acidophilus can help reduce the soreness and pain if you chew one to two tablets two to three times a day until the sores heal. You can also eat yogurt; hold the yogurt in your mouth for about thirty seconds before swallowing. Kefir is another good food source of good bacteria like acidophilus.

CATARACTS

A cataract is a clouding of the lens in the eye that causes blurriness or fogginess. Cataracts can occur in one or both eyes, and they are not contagious. Most cataracts are related to aging; in fact, by age eighty, more than fifty percent of Americans have a cataract or have had cataract surgery. Cataracts are also common in people who have diabetes.

What Causes Cataracts?

The lens in the eye focuses light onto the retina, which is at the back of the eye, and it also adjusts the eye's focus, which allows you to see objects clearly both close up and far away. As we age, the protein in the lens can stick together and form a cloudy area, or cataract. Over time, the cataract may grow and cause more cloudiness. Other symptoms include poor night vision, double vision, fading colors, and seeing a halo around lights, especially at night when driving.

Experts suspect the change in the protein is the result of natural wear and tear on the eye. However, smoking and diabetes also appear to be contributing factors, as well as not protecting the eyes from ultraviolet light.

How Foods and Supplements Can Help

If you want to help prevent cataracts and have better eye health, head toward the kitchen. High on the list are foods rich in vitamin C, as studies show that this antioxidant helps prevent cataracts. So enjoy apricots, asparagus, bell peppers, blueberries, broccoli, cantaloupe, cauliflower, cabbage, grapefruit, greens, guava, lemons, mango, onions, papaya, parsley, peaches, peas, pumpkin, strawberries, sweet potatoes, tangerines, tomatoes, watermelon as much as possible. A vitamin C supplement with bioflavonoids (1,000 mg daily) is also suggested.

Vitamin E (400–800 IU daily) and the mineral selenium (200–300 mcg/day) also help prevent cataracts. Vitamin E is found in almonds, broccoli, Brussel sprouts, greens, seeds, and wheat germ oil. Generally, good sources of selenium include brown rice, eggs, oatmeal, tuna, turkey, and walnuts. Some experts also recommend supplementing with beta-carotene (10,000 IU daily; foods include apricots, cantaloupe, carrots, greens, mango, oatmeal, papaya, peaches, peas, pumpkin, sweet potatoes, tomatoes) and/or riboflavin (10–50 mg/day; foods include broccoli, chicken, fortified cereals, greens, nonfat milk, sweet potato, yogurt) to help treat or slow progression of the disease.

CHRONIC FATIGUE SYNDROME

Imagine feeling so overwhelmingly tired that you can barely get out of bed in the morning. Imagine feeling that way every day. Such fatigue is the hallmark of chronic fatigue syndrome (CFS), a complex and often debilitating condition that affects the brain and various systems throughout the body. Along with the fatigue, people with CFS often experience impaired memory, muscle and joint pain, sleep problems, depression, and vertigo. The Centers for Disease Control and Prevention (CDC) reports that about one million Americans have CFS, and that it affects about four times more women than men. Children and adolescents also get CFS.

What Causes Chronic Fatigue Syndrome?

Chronic fatigue syndrome is a very complex disorder, and so far researchers have not definitively identified its cause. They have, however, identified probable candidates and triggers, including chronic viral infection, inflammation, chemical and/or metal sensitivities, nutritional deficiencies, food intolerances, extreme emotional or physical stress, thyroid deficiency, abnormal responses by the immune system to stressors, and excessive levels of free radicals (oxidative stress). Most likely the cause of chronic fatigue syndrome is a combination of these and other factors, including genetics.

How Foods and Supplements Can Help

Various foods and supplements can help relieve some of the symptoms of chronic fatigue syndrome. Omega-3 fatty acids, for example, relieve inflammation that is characteristic of CFS. Be sure to include avocados, Brazil nuts, flaxseed, salmon, sardines, tuna, and walnuts in your diet. A fish oil supplement (1,000 mg daily) is also recommended. A recent Belgian study found that zinc may be helpful in alleviating symptoms of chronic fatigue syndrome. Foods that provide zinc include asparagus, calf's liver, greens, peas, pumpkin seeds, sesame seeds, and yogurt. Supplemental zinc (15–30 mg daily) is suggested.

Coenzyme Q10 (200–400 mg per day taken in divided doses) is involved in energy production, so this supplement may increase your energy level. It may also relieve the muscle pain and weakness associated with CFS. Magnesium can help muscles relax and enhance energy production. A suggested dose is 200 mg three times daily, which should be balanced with twice the amount of calcium to counter the mineral's laxative effects. Magnesium-rich foods include almonds, avocado, beans (dried), greens, peas, pumpkin seeds, tofu.

COMMON COLD

It's rare to find someone who has not experienced the common cold: more than one billion cases of this viral infection occur each year in the United States, and children typically get between three and eight colds per year. The common cold is responsible for more lost days of school and work than any other illness. Although colds can develop at any time, they emerge most often during the winter months and/or during a rainy season.

What Causes the Common Cold?

More than two hundred different viruses can cause a cold. Once the virus takes hold, people are most contagious during days two and three of their illness, and are usually not contagious by days seven to ten. Symptoms include sneezing, runny nose, and nasal congestion, and may be accompanied by headache, sore throat, cough, or muscle aches. Adults seldom develop a fever, but young children often do.

How Foods and Supplements Can Help

The debate continues: can vitamin C help prevent the common cold, reduce the severity of symptoms, and/or reduce how long you have a cold? Dozens of studies make claims on both sides of the argument. For now, the bottom line is this: vitamin C supplements (500–1,000 mg daily) may offer some limited protection, and once a cold takes hold, supplements can do little to reduce the frequency or severity of symptoms.

Adding 50,000 to 100,000 IU of the antioxidant beta-carotene to your daily supplement schedule can boost your immune system against this common viral infection. Foods rich in these potent antioxidants should also be a regular part of your diet: apricots, asparagus, bell peppers, blueberries, broccoli, cantaloupe, cauliflower, cabbage, grapefruit, greens, guava, lemons, mango, onions, papaya, parsley, peaches, peas, pumpkin, strawberries, sweet potatoes, tangerines, tomatoes, and watermelon.

Zinc lozenges may reduce both the severity and duration of symptoms. Lozenges that contain about 3.3 mg of elemental zinc each should be taken every two hours during the day immediately after the symptoms appear and stopped as soon as symptoms disappear. Long-term use of this high level of zinc can lead to a copper deficiency, so use them only while you have a cold.

Garlic not only wards off vampires, it can chase the common cold as well. Volunteers who took a garlic supplement daily for twelve weeks were significantly less likely to get a cold and, if they did, they had much less severe symptoms and were ill for a much briefer time. You can take a garlic supplement (equal to 2,500 mg of fresh garlic daily) or include two to three cloves in your daily diet. Another approach is to take probiotics (2–3 billion CFUs [colony-forming units] daily of a supplement that contains three or more species), which can reduce the duration and severity of common cold episodes. The addition of yogurt to your diet is also helpful.

CONSTIPATION

In conventional medical circles, constipation is defined as having a bowel movement less than three times a week, with stools that are hard, dry, and/or difficult to pass. Within a broader medical community (naturopaths, alternative practitioners), many believe daily bowel movements should be considered the norm. In either case, the American College of

Gastroenterology reports that about 4.5 million Americans a year report having frequent constipation and another 45 million suffer with it occasionally. Women and people older than sixty-five are most likely to experience constipation.

What Causes Constipation?

The most common cause of constipation is a low-fiber diet, as most Americans do not consume the recommended amount of dietary fiber (see "Fiber"). Other factors that can contribute to constipation include lack of exercise, use of certain medications or supplements (e.g., iron supplements, narcotics, diuretics, calcium channel blockers), intestinal diseases (e.g., irritable bowel syndrome, Crohn's disease), milk, dehydration, abuse of laxatives, or a change in lifestyle or habits (e.g., traveling, emotional stress, surgery).

How Foods and Supplements Can Help

Foods high in fiber should be at the top of your list to prevent or treat constipation. Include as many of these foods as you can in your diet: apples, barley, beans (dried, cooked), broccoli, brown rice, carrots, flaxseed, lentils, oats, oranges, pears, peas, squash, whole grains, and 100% bran cereals. Another food-related treatment for constipation is **probiotics**— good bacteria—found in yogurt and kefir, and available in supplements as well. Consider taking 16 billion CFUs of a mixed probiotics supplement with each meal for three to four days, then reduce the dose to 11 billion CFUs for another three days, then stay at 2 billion as a maintenance dose to help keep your intestinal tract healthy. One more simple approach that many people forget to do: drink water. Drinking six or more eight-ounce glasses of water daily is especially important when you eat fiber and if you have constipation.

DEPRESSION

Depression is an illness that affects the mind as well as the body. More than a temporary bout of sadness, it is a pervasive, chronic condition that involves intense or deep emotions that have a negative impact on how people feel about themselves, their circumstances, and their life.

Of the different types of depressive disorder, one of the most common is major depression. Symptoms can vary in severity and duration, and generally include several or more of the following:

- Persistent feelings of sadness, anxiety, or "emptiness"
- Feelings of hopelessness, guilt, worthlessness, and/or helplessness
- Loss of interest or pleasure in activities once enjoyed, including sex
- Fatigue
- Problems with concentration, memory, and decision-making
- Sleep problems
- Thoughts of suicide and/or suicidal attempts
- Irritability, restlessness
- Changes in appetite and/or weight

What Causes Depression?

Depression tends to run in families, which suggests that the susceptibility is inherited. Emotionally charged circumstances, such as death, divorce, unemployment, and financial worries can trigger depression. Hormonal changes, especially those experienced by women around menstruation, pregnancy, premenopause, and menopause, are factors. Research shows that the brain undergoes chemical changes in people who are depressed, and this information is helpful because it gives experts tangible ways to approach prevention and treatment. Food and nutritional supplements are some of those ways.

How Foods and Supplements Can Help

It's a fact: food affects mood. The brain chemical serotonin, a key player in depression, needs many nutrients to operate efficiently, and one major nutrient is vitamin B-6. People who are depressed often have low levels of both B-6 and serotonin, a situation that may be worsened by the use of oral contraceptives or hormone replacement therapy. Therefore B-6 supplements (25–100 mg daily) and B-6–rich foods (e.g., asparagus, bananas, bell peppers, cabbage, carrots, cauliflower, celery, garlic, greens, squash, tomato, tuna, turmeric, watermelon) are recommended.

Low levels of folate are associated with depression and can also interfere with the effectiveness of certain antidepressant drugs (selective serotonin reuptake inhibitors). Folic acid supplements (400–800 mcg daily) and foods with good levels of the vitamin (e.g., asparagus, avocado, beans (dried), beets, bell peppers, broccoli, cabbage, cauliflower, corn, fortified cereals, greens, oranges, papaya, parsnips, peas, soybeans, tofu, turkey, wheat germ) are suggested.

An omega-3 deficiency often is associated with low serotonin levels. Supplements (1,000 mg EPA and DHA daily) plus foods such as avocados, Brazil nuts, flaxseed, salmon, sardines, tuna, and walnuts, can be beneficial. Low levels of vitamin D also have been implicated in depression. A 400 IU supplement taken daily, along with foods that provide the vitamin (e.g., cod liver oil, eggs, fortified cereals and nonfat milk, salmon), are recommended.

DIABETES

Diabetes is an endocrine disorder in which the body does not produce insulin (type 1 diabetes; about 5% of all cases), or the insulin it does produce is insufficient or the body cannot utilize it properly (type 2 diabetes; more than 90% of all cases). Insulin is needed to convert sugar, starches, and other food components into energy that the body must have to function. Insulin is necessary for life.

More than twenty million Americans have diabetes and more than twice that number are at risk for the disease. Because diabetes is associated with many serious complications, including heart disease, blindness, kidney failure, gangrene, and neuropathy (nerve damage), it is critical to take steps to prevent and properly treat this disease.

What Causes Diabetes?

Type 1 diabetes appears in childhood or adolescence and is believed to be an autoimmune disease, which means the body attacks its own healthy cells (the pancreas, which produces insulin). Genetics may also play a part. Type 2 diabetes usually develops in people age forty and older, although cases are occurring in much younger people today. Risk factors for type 2 diabetes include obesity/overweight, high blood pressure, high cholesterol, high triglycerides, smoking, sedentary lifestyle, and a high-fat diet.

In healthy people, insulin helps glucose (sugar) enter the cells and provide energy for life. When insulin production or use is faulty, glucose stays in the blood and damages blood vessels and organs throughout the body. Therefore people with diabetes need to regulate their blood glucose levels either by taking insulin (type 1) or by diet, exercise, and/or medication (type 2).

How Foods and Supplements Can Help

In most people who are at risk for or who have type 2 diabetes, proper diet and exercise can prevent or reverse the disease. In addition to a diet that emphasizes fresh fruits and vegetables, whole grains and legumes, and high-quality protein as a way to both lose weight and prevent or manage diabetes, some supplements and specific foods may be beneficial. Low levels of magnesium, for example, are associated with poor blood sugar control and the development of diabetic complications. Supplementing magnesium (250–500 mg daily) plus eating foods high in magnesium (e.g., almonds, avocado, beans [dried], greens, peas, pumpkin seeds, tofu) can help.

Coenzyme Q10 assists with carbohydrate metabolism and offers protection against diabetic complications. A supplement (120 mg daily) may help; food sources of CoQ10 include broccoli, eggs, red meat, spinach, wheat germ, and whole grains. Supplemental vitamin E (400 IU daily) may improve glycemic control and help prevent complications of diabetes, and you should include food sources of vitamin E daily as well (e.g., almonds, broccoli, greens, kiwi, mango, peanut butter, sunflower seeds, wheat germ oil). Another helpful substance is garlic, which appears to have antidiabetic properties and the ability to help prevent diabetic complications. Take a supplement that provides a dose that equals 2,500 mg of fresh (two cloves of fresh garlic) daily, or include two cloves of fresh garlic in your diet daily. Odor-free supplements are available.

DIARRHEA

Nearly one hundred million adults and millions of children experience diarrhea in the United States each year. Characterized by loose, watery stools, bloating, and pressure in the intestinal area, diarrhea is second only to the common cold when it comes to causing lost days at work and school. Most cases are minor and can be treated easily at home without a doctor's care.

What Causes Diarrhea?

Viral infections are the cause of the majority of diarrhea cases. Symptoms are usually mild to moderate, may include a low-grade fever, and generally last from three to seven days. Some common viruses that cause diarrhea include rotavirus (common in infants), Norwalk virus, and adenovirus. Diarrhea caused by bacterial infections is usually related to food poisoning. Symptoms are typically more severe and often include vomiting, severe stomach cramps, and frequent diarrhea. Diarrhea can quickly cause dehydration, especially in young children and the elderly, so it is important to drink water throughout the day.

How Foods and Supplements Can Help

One of the best supplements to help heal your intestinal tract when you have diarrhea is probiotics, especially supplements that contain *Lactobacilli acidophilus, L. ramnosus GG,*

L. casei, and *Bifidobacteria* spp. Take a probiotics supplement that contains at least three different species of good bacteria: take 16 billion CFUs per meal for three to four days, then 11 billion CFUs for an additional three to four days, then stay on a maintenance dose of 2 billion CFUs to help keep your intestinal tract healthy.

Green tea (decaffeinated) provides antioxidants to help fight the infection that causes diarrhea, and helps replace lost fluids as well. Electrolytes (e.g., sodium, potassium) lost during a bout of diarrhea can be replaced by including bananas, orange juice, and vegetable juice in your diet. Foods that are easy to digest, low in fat, low in fiber, and/or that contain pectin (which helps solidify stool) are best to eat when you have diarrhea, including applesauce, apples, bananas, beets (cooked), brown rice, carrots (cooked), grapefruit, and toast. Blueberries have long been used to treat diarrhea because they contain tannins, which firm up loose stool.

DIVERTICULOSIS/DIVERTICULITIS

Diverticulosis is a condition in which tiny sacs called diverticula develop in the colon (large intestine) and push out from the colon walls. If the diverticula become infected and burst, abdominal pain, fever, and tenderness result, and the condition is then called diverticulitis.

Diverticular disease is common in the Western world but rare in Africa and Asia. More than fifty percent of people older than sixty in the United States have diverticular disease.

What Causes Diverticulosis/Diverticulitis?

The walls of the colon thicken with age. Over time, pressure on the walls from the passage of feces, especially if constipation or hard stools occurred frequently, can cause the inner intestinal lining to push out through any openings in the walls (herniate) and form diverticula. Most people who have diverticulosis are unaware they have the disease because they have no symptoms: only twenty percent of people with diverticulosis develop symptoms, which can include diarrhea, bloating, stomach cramps, and constipation. If the diverticula become infected and burst, the result is diverticulitis.

How Foods and Supplements Can Help

The best approach is prevention: eat a high-fiber diet (see "Fiber), drink enough water, and avoid straining when eliminating. Some excellent high-fiber foods include barley, beans (dried), brown rice, bulgar, figs (dried), lentils, peas, sweet potatoes, and whole grains. Other good sources include apples, apricots, beets, broccoli, cabbage, cauliflower, greens, papaya, pears, and whole grains.

Probiotic supplements, along with yogurt and kefir, can provide the beneficial bacteria that can help heal the intestinal tract. If you experience symptoms of diverticulitis, a suggested dose of probiotics (choose a supplement that contains at least four different species) is 10 to 15 billion CFUs per meal until your symptoms improve, then 5 to 6 billion daily for a week, then 2 billion daily to help maintain a healthy colon.

EAR INFECTIONS

Ear infections are the second most common illness that affects infants and young children in the United States. Seventy-five percent of children have at least one ear infection by the time they are three years old. Although there are several types of ear infections, the most common is acute otitis media, or a middle ear infection. Acute otitis media is characterized by fluid in the middle ear, pain, a red eardrum, and in some patients, fever. In chronic cases, the fluid remains in the ear for six weeks or longer.

What Causes Ear Infections?

In children, ear infections are especially common for several reasons. The eustachian tube, the passageway that connects the middle ear to the back of the throat, allows mucus to drain out of the middle ear into the throat and also equalizes the air pressure in the middle ear to the outside pressure. If the tube becomes irritated or blocked by congestion, fluid can build up in the middle ear and become trapped. Any viruses or bacteria that also become trapped can breed and eventually cause an ear infection. Another reason is that the immune system does not fully develop until age seven, which means young children are more susceptible to infections. One more cause is partial blockage of the eustachian tube opening by the adenoids (the glands located in the back of the upper throat near the eustachian tubes). Exposure to cigarette smoke and bottle feeding are also risk factors for ear infections.

How Foods and Supplements Can Help

Prevention of ear infections is your first step: make sure your children (and you!) eat foods rich in antioxidants, especially vitamin A/beta-carotene (e.g., apricots, cantaloupe, carrots, greens, mango, oatmeal, papaya, peaches, peas, pumpkin, sweet potatoes, tomatoes) and vitamin C (e.g., all those mentioned, plus asparagus, bell peppers, blueberries, broccoli, cabbage, cauliflower, grapefruit, guava, lemons, onions, papaya, parsley, peaches, peas, strawberries, watermelon). These vitamins, along with zinc (food sources include beans, brown rice, fortified cereals, lentils, oatmeal, oysters, peas, salmon, yogurt), are potent immune system boosters. Children who do not get enough of these important nutrients may need a supplement; talk to your doctor about the most appropriate multivitamin/mineral supplement for your child.

Probiotics may help reduce the incidence of ear infections. Chewable probiotic supplements are available for children, and the contents of capsules can be mixed with formula or water for infants or children who cannot chew tablets. The suggested dose for children younger than 10 years is 500 million to 1 billion CFUs daily. If your child gets an ear infection and takes antibiotics, use of probiotics is especially critical to help prevent yeast and other infections that can occur with antibiotic use. The suggested dose, both during and for several weeks after antibiotic use, is 2 billion CFUs daily for children younger than 10 years.

ECZEMA

Eczema, or dermatitis, is a common inflammatory allergic condition of the skin that can affect people of any age. Up to twenty percent of children develop eczema, and it typically first appears before the age of five years. In contrast, only one to two percent of adults have the disease. For some people with eczema, the disease improves over time, while for others the condition is chronic or recurrent.

What Causes Eczema?

Eczema is believed to be caused by a combination of genetic and environmental factors. An allergy to certain irritants and allergens (e.g., pollen, molds, certain foods, food preservatives, detergents, synthetic fibers) can cause eczema in susceptible individuals. Symptoms of eczema include dry, extremely itchy skin, oozing blisters, and dry, leathery skin that has an abnormal amount of pigment. Environmental factors such as temperature changes, exposure to water, and stress can make symptoms worse. It is not unusual for people with eczema to scratch their skin until it bleeds.

How Foods and Supplements Can Help

Nutrients that promote skin health and new cell formation, and that can help ward off free-radical damage and inflammation are the cornerstones of prevention and treatment. This fight involves bringing in the antioxidant vitamins A, C, and E, and selenium: vitamin A helps with new cells, C strengthens the skin, E promotes skin healing, and selenium is a key player in the entire antioxidant process. Suggested dosages are vitamin A/beta-carotene, 5,000–10,000 IU/day; vitamin C, 1,000 mg twice daily; vitamin E, 400 IU/day; selenium, 50–200 mcg/day. Some of the foods that provide good amounts of these antioxidants include (for vitamins A/beta-carotene and C): apricots, asparagus, bell peppers, blueberries, broccoli, cabbage, cantaloupe, carrots, cauliflower, grapefruit, greens, guava, lemons, mango, onions, papaya, parsley, peaches, peas, pumpkin, strawberries, sweet potatoes, tangerines, tomatoes, watermelon; (vitamin E): almonds, broccoli, greens, kiwi, mango, peanut butter, sunflower seeds, wheat germ oil; and (selenium): brown rice, eggs, oatmeal, tuna, turkey, walnuts.

Although all the B vitamins participate in maintaining skin health (including helping oil-producing glands keep the skin moist and smooth), vitamin B-6 (pyridoxine) is especially associated with dermatitis because it is key in regenerating new skin cells. Suggested supplement dosage is 50 to 100 mg/day. Foods that contain good levels of B-6 include asparagus, bananas, bell peppers, cabbage, carrots, cauliflower, celery, garlic, greens, squash, tomatoes, tuna, turmeric, and watermelon.

Studies show that probiotics also can help prevent eczema in children. Look for supplements that contain *Lactobacilli ramnosus GG,* and discuss the most appropriate dose with your physician.

FIBROCYSTIC BREAST CHANGES

Fibrocystic breast is a common, benign (noncancerous) condition in which tender, sometimes painful lumps develop in one or both breasts. This condition affects more than sixty percent of women and occurs most often in women between the ages of thirty and fifty. Some women experience constant or near constant discomfort or pain, while others have little or no pain.

At one time, this condition was called a disease, but the presence of benign breast lumps in women is very common and is not a disease. Fibrocystic breast changes is also known as mammary dysplasia, chronic cystic mastitis, and benign breast disease.

What Causes Fibrocystic Breast Changes?

Fluctuations in hormone activity are the most significant factor in the cause of fibrocystic breast. Estrogen and progesterone cause cells in the breast to grow and multiply, while other hormones (e.g., growth hormone, thyroid, prolactin, insulin) also affect breast cells. Together these hormones stimulate breast tissue growth. Eventually the cells in the breast break down as part of their natural life cycle, but they leave behind cell fragments. These fragments and any inflammation that usually occurs can cause scarring of the ducts in the breast. The amount of inflammation, scarring, and cell breakdown varies from woman to woman and can fluctuate from month to month.

How Foods and Supplements Can Help

The value of foods and supplements in relieving symptoms of fibrocystic breast condition is still under investigation, but there have been many anecdotal reports of success. Vitamin E, for example, may relieve inflammation and increase metabolism of female hormones. Susan M. Lark, MD, a physician specializing in women's health and author of *The PMS Self-Help Book*, recommends taking 600 IU of vitamin E daily to help with fibrocystic breast symptoms. Excess estrogen is a contributing factor for fibrocystic breast, and dietary fiber can help eliminate estrogen from the body. Therefore, including high-fiber foods in your diet may help relieve your symptoms. Some choices include barley, beans (dried), brown rice, bulgar, figs (dried), lentils, peas, sweet potatoes, and whole grains. Other good sources include apples, apricots, beets, broccoli, cabbage, cauliflower, greens, papaya, and pears.

Dr. Lark also recommends taking beta-carotene (25,000–50,000 IU daily) to fight symptoms. Carrots and sweet potatoes have very high beta-carotene values; others include apricots, cantaloupe, greens, mango, oatmeal, papaya, peaches, peas, pumpkin, and tomatoes. Vitamin B-6 may be effective because it is known to help maintain normal hormone levels. A supplement of 50 mg two to three times daily may help reduce breast pain and tenderness. Foods that contain B-6 include asparagus, bananas, bell peppers, cabbage, carrots, cauliflower, celery, garlic, greens, squash, tomato, tuna, turmeric, and watermelon.

FIBROMYALGIA

Fibromyalgia is a chronic condition whose most characteristic symptoms are widespread chronic pain and muscle tenderness, overwhelming fatigue, and sleep problems. The pain and tenderness typically affect the neck, back, shoulders, pelvic area, and hands, but can involve any part of the body. Other symptoms may include rash, headache, irritable bowel syndrome, memory problems, depression, dizziness, cold hands and/or feet, and neurological problems. Approximately three to six percent of people in the United States have fibromyalgia. Although it mostly affects women, it also strikes men and children.

What Causes Fibromyalgia?

Experts are still searching for the causes of fibromyalgia, but it appears the pain is related to a dysfunction in the central nervous system that interprets pain perception. Genetic factors also may predispose people to be highly susceptible to the disease. Some people with fibromyalgia, for example, develop symptoms after experiencing a triggering event, such as an injury, illness, or surgery.

How Foods and Supplements Can Help

Since inflammation is a major cause of the pain and tenderness associated with fibromyalgia, choose foods and nutrients that fight it. One potent anti-inflammatory substance is omega-3 fatty acids. When you include flaxseed and flaxseed oil in your diet, for example, the body converts the ALA (alpha linolenic acid) in flaxseed into prostaglandins, which are anti-inflammatory agents. Other dietary sources of omega-3s, including salmon, tuna, and walnuts, contain oils that need no conversion to do their anti-inflammatory work. Supplementation with omega-3 fatty acids (1,000 mg EPA plus DHA daily) is also recommended.

Magnesium along with malic acid can greatly improve energy and fatigue. Supplementation with 100 to 200 mg of magnesium and 400 to 800 mg of malic acid three times daily, twenty minutes before each meal, is suggested. (If you have kidney or heart problems, talk to your doctor before taking magnesium supplements.)

A diet that focuses on foods rich in antioxidants—especially vitamin A/beta-carotene, vitamin C, vitamin E, and selenium—is recommended because antioxidants fight free radicals, which cause inflammation. Some of the foods that contain one or more of these potent antioxidants are almonds (vitamin E), apricots, asparagus, bell peppers, blueberries, broccoli, brown rice (selenium), cabbage, cantaloupe, carrots, cauliflower, eggs (selenium), grapefruit, greens, guava, lemons, mango, oatmeal, onions, papaya, parsley, peaches, peas, pumpkin, strawberries, sunflower seeds (vitamin E), sweet potatoes, tangerines, tomatoes, turkey (selenium), walnuts (selenium), watermelon, wheat germ (vitamin E). Supplementation with vitamin A/beta-carotene (5,000–10,000 IU/day), vitamin C (500–1,000 mg daily), vitamin E (400 IU daily), and selenium (100–200 mcg daily) is suggested.

GALLSTONES

Gallstones are solid particles composed of cholesterol, fats, bile salts, proteins, and bilirubin—waste products from the breakdown of blood cells in the liver—that form in the gallbladder. About eighty percent of all gallstones are made primarily of hardened cholesterol; the remaining twenty percent are called pigment stones and are composed mainly of bilirubin.

Gallstones can be as small as a grain of sand or as large as a golf ball, and one or more stones can develop in the gallbladder at any time. Women are twice as likely to develop gallstones as men, and both men and women older than sixty are more susceptible to gallstones than their younger counterparts.

What Causes Gallstones?

Cholesterol stones develop when there is excess cholesterol or bilirubin in the bile, not enough bile salts in the bile, or if the gallbladder is unable to empty properly. Pigment stones are usually seen in people who have biliary tract infections, cirrhosis, or hereditary blood disorders. What experts do not know for certain, however, is why any of these situations that result in gallstones develop in the first place.

You may be at greater risk of developing gallstones if you are a woman, have a family history of gallstones, eat a high-fat and/or low-fiber diet, are overweight, take cholesterol-lowering drugs, have diabetes, are older than sixty, and/or have experienced rapid weight loss. Native Americans are at especially high risk of the disease.

How Foods and Supplements Can Help

To prevent the development of gallstone, follow a low-fat diet. Adequate fiber from fruits, vegetables, whole grains, and legumes is important (e.g., apples, barley, beans (dried, cooked), broccoli, brown rice, carrots, lentils, pears, peas, squash, whole grains, 100% bran cereals), especially gel-forming fibers found in flaxseed, oat bran, and pectin (found in fruits). Drink at least six eight-ounce glasses of water daily to maintain the proper water content of bile.

You can promote bile production by eating radishes (two to four per day) as well as taking supplements of vitamin C (1,000 mg two to three times daily) and vitamin E (400 to 800 IU daily). Also include foods rich in vitamin C (e.g., apricots, asparagus, bell peppers, blueberries, broccoli, cabbage, cantaloupe, cauliflower, grapefruit, greens, guava, lemons, mango, onions, papaya, parsley, peaches, peas, pumpkin, strawberries, sweet potatoes, tangerines, tomatoes, watermelon) and vitamin E (e.g., almonds, broccoli, greens, kiwi, mango, peanut butter, sunflower seeds, wheat germ oil).

GINGIVITIS

Gingivitis means "inflammation of the gums" (gingival). This very common gum (periodontal) disease can develop in children as young as three years old. By adolescence, gingivitis is estimated to affect between seventy and ninety percent of teens, and the Food and Drug Administration reports that about seventy-five percent of adults have gum disease. During the early stages of gingivitis, many people do not experience pain and don't notice the disease until a more serious form of periodontal disease develops.

What Causes Gingivitis?

The main cause of gingivitis is poor dental hygiene. A buildup of plaque—sticky material composed of mucus, bacteria, and food particles that attaches itself to the exposed part of your teeth—is the major cause of tooth decay. If plaque is not removed regularly, it transforms into a hard substance called tartar. The plaque and tartar together can irritate the gums, leaving them red, swollen, tender, and susceptible to bleeding.

Other causes of gingivitis can include overly vigorous brushing or flossing of the teeth, uncontrolled diabetes, poorly fitted dentures, braces, or bridges, or misaligned teeth. Left untreated, gingivitis can develop into a more serious dental disease, called periodontitis, in which abscesses may form and teeth can loosen and fall out.

How Foods and Supplements Can Help

If you apply a liquid form of the antioxidant CoQ10 to gums affected by gingivitis, the infection should subside. Taking an oral form of the enzyme (60–120 mg twice daily, gel-cap form preferred) may also eliminate the infection. Vitamin C is critical for healthy gums; take 1,000 mg daily for prevention and 3,000 mg (in three divided doses) daily as treatment, along with eating foods rich in the vitamin, including apricots, asparagus, bell peppers, blueberries, broccoli, cabbage, cantaloupe, cauliflower, grapefruit, greens, guava, lemons, mango, onions, papaya, parsley, peaches, peas, pumpkin, strawberries, sweet potatoes, tangerines, tomatoes, watermelon.

Cranberries contain a compound called proanthocyanidin, which can prevent bacteria from sticking to your gums and teeth. Eating ¼ cup of fresh or frozen (unsweetened) cranberries or drinking three ounces of unsweetened cranberry juice several times a week can help prevent or treat gingivitis.

Green tea contains a class of antioxidants called catechins, which fight oral plaque and bacteria. Drinking several cups of green tea daily can be beneficial, but rinsing your mouth and brushing your teeth with green tea extract daily can also significantly prevent and reduce plaque buildup and kill harmful bacteria.

GLAUCOMA

Glaucoma is an eye disease in which the primary nerve responsible for vision—the optic nerve—is damaged, which causes a loss of sight. Generally, side vision is the first to be affected, and if glaucoma is not treated, central vision loss and blindness can result.

An estimated three million Americans have glaucoma, yet as many as fifty percent are not aware they have the disease because it does not cause symptoms during the early stages, and the loss of side vision is hardly noticeable. It typically affects people age sixty-five and older, and is the leading cause of irreversible blindness around the world.

What Causes Glaucoma?

The front of the eye is filled with fluid that provides the eye with nutrients. This fluid is constantly being produced and drained through a system of meshwork. If the meshwork becomes blocked, pressure can build up in the eye (intraocular pressure) and damage the optic nerve. This is what occurs with the most common type of glaucoma, chronic open-angle glaucoma. The meshwork can clog due to normal aging, which reduces the ability of the eye to drain and thus increases intraocular pressure. Other causes of chronic open-angle glaucoma can include low levels of nitric oxide, genetics, and brain chemical abnormalities.

Normal pressure glaucoma, which is less common, is believed to be caused by decreased blood flow to the optic nerve. Both open-angle and normal pressure glaucoma are painless. Closed-angle glaucoma, which is relatively rare, occurs suddenly and is accompanied by severe eye pain, headache, vomiting, edema, and blurry vision.

How Foods and Supplements Can Help

If you have glaucoma or want to prevent it, eat to keep your intraocular pressure in a normal range. Several nutrients can help you achieve this goal. Magnesium, as a supplement (200–600 mg daily) and/or in certain foods (almonds, avocado, beans (dried), greens, peas, pumpkin seeds, tofu) is important. Vitamin C reportedly reduces intraocular pressure as well. Supplement with 500 to 1,000 mg daily and enjoy vitamin C–rich foods; e.g., apricots, asparagus, bell peppers, blueberries, broccoli, cabbage, cantaloupe, cauliflower, grapefruit, greens, guava, lemons, mango, onions, papaya, parsley, peaches, peas, pumpkin, strawberries, sweet potatoes, tangerines, tomatoes, watermelon.

Yet another helpful nutrient is omega-3 fatty acids, found in avocados, Brazil nuts, flaxseed, salmon, sardines, tuna, and walnuts. Supplement at 1,000 mg of EPA and DHA daily. Lutein, a potent antioxidant and phytonutrient, protects the interior of the eye against free-radical damage. It is found in asparagus, bell peppers, broccoli, carrots, celery, corn, greens, parsley, peas, pumpkin, and squash, and the suggested supplement dose is 6 mg daily.

HEADACHE AND MIGRAINE

Headache is pain behind the head, in the back of the upper neck, or above the eyes or ears, that can be caused by a variety of factors. Generally, headache falls into one of two main categories: primary or secondary. Primary headaches are not associated with other diseases and include tension and migraine headache; secondary headaches are symptoms of other medical ailments. Tension headache is the most common type of headache; at least ninety percent of Americans can expect to experience at least one tension headache during their lifetime. Migraines are typically more severe than tension headache and affect about six percent of men and eighteen percent of women.

Migraine is a moderate to severe headache that may be preceded or accompanied by sensory warnings, such as tingling in the arms or legs, flashing lights, or blind spots. The head pain, which can be debilitating, may also be accompanied by nausea, vomiting, or extreme sensitivity to sound and light. The pain is typically throbbing or pulsating, affects one side of the head only, and increases with physical activity.

What Causes Headache and Migraine?

Tension headaches are appropriately named, as they appear to be triggered by stress, which in turn causes muscle contractions and tension throughout the body. The pain usually begins at the back of the head or base of the neck, where muscles are often tense and thus contribute to the head pain. Another common location for tension headache is the area above the eyes and circling the head.

For migraine, hormone imbalance appears to be a major cause, especially in women, who are much more prone to migraine than men. Factors such as certain foods (e.g., chocolate, alcohol, marinated items), weather changes, emotional stress, sleep difficulties, and some medications can trigger a migraine attack. Pain occurs because the blood vessels dilate (enlarge) and chemicals are released from nerve fibers that encircle the blood vessels. These chemicals cause inflammation and pain.

How Foods and Supplements Can Help

In some cases *eliminating* certain foods can help headaches. It is not unusual for specific foods to trigger headache or migraine, and if you suspect your headaches may be diet related, consult a health-care professional about food allergy testing or doing a food elimination program to uncover which foods may be triggering your head pain. You can also do a food elimination diet on your own.

Foods and nutrients that can help relieve headache and migraine include magnesium, which tends to be in short supply in people who have migraine. Studies suggest that magnesium supplements may reduce the duration of a migraine attack.

Good food sources of magnesium include almonds, avocado, beans (dried), greens, peas, pumpkin seeds, and tofu.

One study found that riboflavin alone (400 mg daily) significantly reduced migraine frequency and the need for antimigraine drugs. Foods that provide a good amount of riboflavin include almonds, eggs, low-fat milk, spinach, and yogurt. Another effective supplement for migraine is CoQ10. Studies show that 100 mg of CoQ10 three times daily significantly reduced the frequency and duration of migraine episodes.

HEART ATTACK

Heart attack, or myocardial infarction, occurs when the blood supply to a part of the heart is blocked. If the flow is not restored quickly, heart muscle cells begin to die from lack of oxygen. Common symptoms of heart attack include chest pain or discomfort (often described as a tight, squeezed, or full feeling in the chest) that may linger or come and go, shortness of breath, and discomfort in the neck, jaw, back, stomach, and one or both arms. Other symptoms that may accompany these include nausea, vomiting, sweating, and fainting.

Approximately 1.1 million heart attacks occur each year in the United States, and about half of the people die. Heart attack is the leading cause of death of both men and women in the United States.

What Causes Heart Attack?

Most heart attacks occur as a result of coronary artery disease (CAD), a condition in which plaque accumulates on the inside walls of the arteries that supply blood and oxygen to the heart. When a portion of the plaque ruptures, a blood clot forms, and if it becomes large enough, it can partially or completely block the flow of blood to the heart from that artery. A much less common cause of heart attack is a severe tightening of the coronary artery due to a spasm. This type of attack may be caused by emotional stress or pain, exposure to extreme cold, use of certain drugs (e.g., cocaine), or smoking.

How Foods and Supplements Can Help

Because CAD is largely related to diet, you can take steps to prevent both CAD and heart attack. Fiber can reduce cholesterol levels, so foods high in fiber are recommended; e.g., apples, barley, beans (dried, cooked), broccoli, brown rice, carrots, flaxseed, lentils, oats, oranges, pears, peas, squash, whole grains, and 100% bran cereals. To ward off inflammation, a key factor in CAD, make omega-3 fatty acids a regular part of your diet. Avocados, Brazil nuts, flaxseed, salmon, sardines, tuna, and walnuts are good sources; a daily supplement containing 1,000 mg of EPA and DHA daily is also a preventive step.

Although soy itself doesn't help prevent CAD, if you substitute soy protein for animal protein you can improve heart health because soy provides fiber, nutrients, and lower saturated fat than animal protein. Tofu, tempeh, and other soy products are recommended.

Low levels of the carotenoids lutein, zeaxanthin, and beta-cryptoxanthin are associated with increased risk of CAD. To boost your levels of these important phytonutrients, be sure to include asparagus, bell peppers, broccoli, carrots, celery, corn, greens, parsley, peas, pumpkin, and squash in your diet often. The suggested supplement dose is 6 mg daily.

HEARTBURN

If you have heartburn (acid indigestion), your heart won't burn, but you will feel a burning sensation in your chest behind your breastbone and in your throat. This feeling may occur after you eat and last for a few minutes or up to several hours. You may also experience chest pain, difficulty swallowing, or a chronic cough or sore throat. Approximately ten percent of Americans experience heartburn on a daily basis, and thirty percent say it's an occasional problem.

What Causes Heartburn?

Heartburn occurs when a valve called the lower esophageal sphincter, which normally keeps stomach acid in the stomach,

malfunctions—it may open too often or not close properly.
Either of these problems causes stomach acid to reflux or seep
into the esophagus and cause a burning sensation. The sphincter may malfunction if there is too much food or pressure in
the stomach (the latter may be caused by obesity or pregnancy), or in response to foods that cause the sphincter to relax; for example, tomatoes, chocolate, citrus, coffee, garlic,
onions, and peppermint. Foods that are high in fat also can
cause heartburn.

Heartburn is the most common symptom of GERD—
gastroesophageal reflux disease—in which stomach acid or
(occasionally) bile flows into the esophagus. This constant irritation of acid and/or bile can damage the esophagus and
cause inflammation, narrowing of the esophagus, and ulcers.

How Foods and Supplements Can Help

To prevent heartburn, avoid fried and/or spicy foods, caffeine, red meat, alcohol, sugar, and refined items. Foods that are
more alkaline (less acidic) are recommended, including fresh
vegetables and fruits, eggs, tofu, tempeh, turkey, and yogurt.

Probiotics can treat heartburn and prevent its recurrence. To
eliminate symptoms, choose a product that contains at least five
species and take 2.5 to 5.5 billion CFUs daily until symptoms are under control, then take 1 to 2 billion daily to maintain
healthy digestion. Also, follow the food suggestions listed above.

Chewable or liquid calcium supplements may also offer relief. The suggested dose is 250 to 500 mg three times daily. A
combination of supplements may be effective for chronic
heartburn: thiamin (500 mg once daily), vitamin B-5
(1,000 mg twice daily), and choline (500 mg three times daily)
until symptoms disappear.

GENITAL HERPES

Genital herpes is a common viral infection and a sexually
transmitted disease. More than 500,000 Americans are diagnosed with the disease each year. Twenty percent (more than

fifty million people) of American adults have genital herpes, but many of them don't know they have the disease because their symptoms are mild or nonexistent. This is a major reason why the disease spreads so easily.

What Causes Herpes?

Genital herpes is most often caused by herpes simplex virus-2 (HSV-2). The herpes simplex virus-1 can also cause genital herpes, but in most cases it causes mouth and lip sores only. When signs of HSV-2 appear, they usually include one or more blisters on or around the genitals or rectum. Once the blisters break, they leave behind sores that can take several weeks to heal. The virus is released from the sores and can spread the disease to another person during sexual or intimate contact. An infected person can also spread the disease even if there are no sores and the skin does not appear to be broken.

Genital herpes can cause recurrent genital sores and can also increase susceptibility to HIV infection. That's because herpes is a chronic infection that can stay in the body indefinitely and weaken the immune system.

Because there is no cure for herpes, treatment focuses on relieving symptoms, reducing the number of outbreaks, and keeping them under control.

How Foods and Supplements Can Help

The foods you choose can help you control herpes. The amino acid lysine, for example, hinders the herpes virus, while arginine stimulates it. Studies suggest you should focus on foods that contain a greater percentage of lysine than arginine, such as beans (dried), chicken, soybeans, and most fruits and vegetables. Foods high in arginine should be avoided and include chocolate, coconut, oats, peanuts, whole wheat, and white flour.

Foods that contain indole-3-carbinol could prevent the herpes virus from reproducing. Researchers at the Northeastern Ohio Universities College of Medicine found that this phytonutrient was ninety-nine percent effective in preventing the virus from replicating in human cells. Broccoli, brussel sprouts, cabbage, cauliflower, rutabaga, turnips, and other cruciferous vegetables are excellent sources of indole-3-carbinol. It is also available as a supplement: suggested dose is 300 to 400 mg daily.

Garlic's potent antiviral properties are effective against herpes virus. You can choose two to five grams of fresh garlic in your daily fare, or select a garlic supplement that provides 2 to 5 mg of allicin daily (2–5 mg garlic oil, 300–1,000 mg of garlic extract). Odorless garlic supplements are available.

HEMORRHOIDS

About ten million Americans have hemorrhoids, a condition in which the veins around the anus or lower rectum are inflamed and swollen. In fact, hemorrhoids are actually varicose veins that develop inside the anus or under the skin around it. Hemorrhoids are most common among pregnant women and people older than fifty. They are seldom dangerous but they can be painful, and for most people the symptoms usually disappear within a few days, although they can recur. In rare cases, hemorrhoids need to be removed surgically.

What Causes Hemorrhoids?

The most common causes of hemorrhoids are pregnancy and straining to eliminate stool. Hemorrhoids typically disappear soon after mothers give birth. Other causes of hemorrhoids include aging, increased pressure on the veins from sitting, chronic diarrhea or constipation, and anal intercourse.

The typical sign of internal hemorrhoids is bright red blood in the toilet bowl or covering the stool. External hemorrhoids usually appear as a painful lump or swelling around the anus that is the result of a blood clot.

How Foods and Supplements Can Help

A high-fiber diet is the best way to both prevent and treat hemorrhoids. Experts agree you need twenty-five to thirty grams of fiber daily to help prevent hemorrhoids and keep your intestinal tract functioning optimally. Some of the best foods to help you reach that goal are apples, avocado, barley, beans (dried, cooked), broccoli, brown rice, carrots, flaxseed, grapefruit, lentils, oats, oranges, pears, peas, squash, whole grains, and 100% bran cereals. Fiber helps keep your stools soft enough to pass without straining.

Anecdotal reports say that dark berries, such as blueberries and blackberries, help strengthen the walls of the inflamed veins of hemorrhoids and in turn reduce swelling and pain. Experts believe that the phytonutrients anthocyanins and proanthocyanidins are responsible for these benefits.

HIGH CHOLESTEROL

Believe it or not, your body needs cholesterol, so it's a *good* thing to have. But too much of a good thing is *not* good, and that is true of cholesterol. High cholesterol levels in the bloodstream are associated with serious medical conditions, including atherosclerosis, heart attack, and stroke.

A diagnosis of high cholesterol is defined as a value of 240 mg/dL or higher, which places you at high risk for heart attack, stroke, liver failure, and other serious problems. A value less than 200 mg/dL is considered to be healthy. Approximately 107 million adults have cholesterol levels higher than 200 mg/dL, and an additional 38 million have levels greater than 240 mg/dL.

What Causes High Cholesterol?

Cholesterol piggybacks a ride on proteins as it travels through the bloodstream. This cholesterol-protein combination is called a lipoprotein, and there are two main types: low-density lipoprotein (LDL), or bad cholesterol, so named because it accumulates in the arteries and hinders blood flow; and high-density lipoprotein (HDL), or good cholesterol, which gathers excess cholesterol and removes it from the blood.

Certain factors can have a negative impact on LDL and HDL, including inactivity, an unhealthy diet (one high in fats, sugars, and processed foods), being overweight, and smoking. Genetics may also play a part, as you can inherit the tendency for the liver to produce too much cholesterol or for your cells to inadequately remove cholesterol from your blood.

How Foods and Supplements Can Help

If you want to eat your way to better cholesterol levels, you need to significantly reduce your intake of high-fat, high-cholesterol foods. These include red meat, full-fat dairy products, and eggs. Small amounts of skinless chicken and turkey are acceptable. Focus instead on fresh vegetables and fruits (avocados are okay in moderation), whole grains, and beans and legumes.

Some foods can lower cholesterol levels, including fatty fish (salmon, tuna, which are high in omega-3 fatty acids), oat bran, oatmeal, and walnuts, and these foods may be as effective as some cholesterol-lowering medications. Foods high in fiber (e.g., apples, avocado, barley, beans (dried, cooked), broccoli, brown rice, carrots, flaxseed, grapefruit, lentils, oats, oranges, pears, peas, squash, whole grains, and 100% bran cereals) also help reduce cholesterol levels, and eating twenty-five to thirty grams of fiber daily can help you achieve that goal.

Several studies show that green tea reduces total cholesterol and raises HDL cholesterol in people and animals. One study's results indicate that the polyphenols in green tea promote the elimination of cholesterol from the body and also block its absorption. The American Heart Association recommends taking 2 to 4 g of omega-3 fatty acids (EPA and DHA) daily for high cholesterol.

HYPERTENSION

High blood pressure—or hypertension—is a serious condition in which the blood presses against the walls of the blood vessels at an abnormally high level, which places a great burden not only on the vessels but on the heart and other organs as well. This stress puts the affected individuals at great risk for atherosclerosis, heart attack, heart failure, stroke, kidney failure, glaucoma, and other critical medical conditions. In fact, hypertension is the leading cause of stroke and a major cause of heart attack in the United States.

Hypertension is defined in stages: normal blood pressure is less than 120/80 mmHg; prehypertension, 120–139/80–89 mmHg; stage 1, 140–159/90–99 mmHg; and stage 2, 160 and higher/100 mmHg and higher. Approximately eighty million Americans older than sixty years have high blood pressure, and because it is basically a symptomless disease, about one-third are unaware they have it.

What Causes Hypertension?

The exact causes of hypertension are not entirely clear, but many factors can contribute to its development, including smoking, being overweight, inactivity, high salt intake, high-fat diet, high alcohol intake, stress, aging, family history of high blood pressure, chronic kidney disease, and thyroid disorders. High blood pressure that has no apparent cause is called primary, or essential, hypertension, and it is the most common type. It often responds to positive lifestyle changes, such as improved diet, weight loss, and exercise. Secondary hypertension is associated with an organic cause, such as pregnancy or thyroid disease.

How Foods and Supplements Can Help

Avoiding the salt shaker and salty foods can help reduce blood pressure, and you can boost that effort by including high-potassium foods in your diet, including apricots, avocados, bananas, cantaloupe, oranges, prunes, tomatoes, and vegetable juice. Potassium supplements are not recommended.

Some studies indicate that adding low-fat dairy products, such as nonfat milk and yogurt (which contain calcium, potassium, and magnesium) to a diet that already contains lots of fruits and vegetables can reduce blood pressure. Other research shows that taking a calcium supplement (800–1,500 mg daily) can help prevent hypertension related to pregnancy. Omega-3 fatty acids help reduce hypertension, as demonstrated in several studies. Flaxseed, salmon, tuna, and walnuts are good food sources; a suggested supplement dose is 1,000 mg daily.

Antioxidants can also improve hypertension. A 2007 study

published in the *American Journal of Hypertension* reported that people with hypertension who took 1,000 mg of vitamin C and 400 IU of vitamin E daily for eight weeks had a significant improvement in blood flow and arterial stiffness. When researchers in Australia evaluated a dozen studies of the impact of CoQ10 on hypertension, they found that the antioxidant caused a significant decrease in blood pressure in all the studies. A recommended dose is 50 mg twice daily.

HUMAN IMMUNODEFICIENCY VIRUS (HIV)

The human immunodeficiency virus (HIV) is a sexually transmitted disease in which the virus destroys white blood cells (called CD4 lymphocytes) that typically protect the body against disease-causing organisms. As CD4 cells are destroyed, the immune system weakens and makes the body vulnerable to a wide range of infections, diseases, and illnesses. Without treatment, people with HIV can expect to develop acquired immunodeficiency syndrome (AIDS) within eight to ten years. With treatment, it can take up to fifteen years or longer.

According to the Centers for Disease Control and Prevention (CDC), an estimated 1,039,000 to 1,185,000 people in the United States had HIV/AIDS at the end of 2003. Approximately one-quarter of them were undiagnosed or unaware they were infected.

What Causes HIV?

The most common way people are infected with HIV is through sexual contact: vaginal, oral, and/or anal sex, heterosexual or homosexual. The virus is also transmitted through infected blood transfusions, shared needles, accidental needle sticks by health workers, and from infected pregnant women to their infants. Once the virus is in the body, it attaches to CD4 lymphocytes, invades them, and uses the CD4 cells to reproduce. The new copies of the virus enter the bloodstream and attack other cells. As the number of CD4 cells decreases, the immune system weakens.

Some of the first symptoms of HIV include swollen glands, diarrhea, cough, weight loss, fever, and shortness of breath. Over time, these symptoms may increase in severity and others occur, including soaking night sweats, rash, diarrhea, severe chills, headache, weight loss, fatigue, and vision problems.

How Foods and Supplements Can Help

Although there is no cure for HIV or AIDS, certain foods and supplements may help slow progression of the disease and relieve symptoms. A 2004 study published in the *New England Journal of Medicine*, for example, found that progression of HIV slowed in pregnant women who were given a B-complex formula and vitamins C (500 mg) and E (30 mg). The nutrients also delayed the need for medication and significantly reduced symptoms, including fatigue, rash, and gastrointestinal problems. Food sources of these vitamins include (vitamin C): apricots, asparagus, bell peppers, blueberries, broccoli, cabbage, cantaloupe, cauliflower, grapefruit, greens, guava, lemons, mango, onions, papaya, parsley, peaches, peas, pumpkin, strawberries, sweet potatoes, tangerines, tomatoes, and watermelon; (vitamin E) almonds, broccoli, greens, kiwi, mango, peanut butter, sunflower seeds, and wheat germ oil. When it comes to B vitamins, good sources come from every food group, so eat a variety of the foods mentioned in Part I: fruits and vegetables, whole grains, legumes, and fish.

A 2007 study published in the *Archives of Internal Medicine* reported that 200 mcg of selenium taken daily by people with HIV significantly slowed progression of the disease and improved CD4 counts. Sources of selenium include brown rice, eggs, oatmeal, tuna, turkey, and walnuts; lesser amounts can be found in fruits and vegetables.

INFERTILITY (MEN)

Infertility is the inability to achieve pregnancy after one year of unprotected sexual intercourse. According to the National Institutes of Health, male infertility is a factor in approximately forty percent of the 2.6 million infertile married couples in the United States. One-half of these men cannot father children, and a small percentage have a treatable medical condition.

What Causes Male Infertility?

Male infertility can be the result of impaired sperm mobility, impaired sperm production, and a deficiency of testosterone. These problems can be caused by a number of factors, including a varicocele (when veins in the scrotum are dilated, which warms the scrotum and affects sperm production), hormone dysfunction, illness (e.g., sexually transmitted disease, high fever, infection, kidney disease, testicular cancer), medications (e.g., those used to treat arthritis or high blood pressure), injury or trauma to the reproductive system, or obstruction of the reproductive tract. Any of these factors can temporarily or permanently affect sperm levels and/or viability and prevent conception.

How Foods and Supplements Can Help

The phytonutrient lycopene may improve male infertility, according to a recent study of fifty men who had low sperm counts. After the men took lycopene supplements (2000 mcg) twice daily for three months, sixty-six percent had an increase in sperm concentration and fifty-three percent had an increase in sperm motility. Food sources of lycopene include asparagus, bell peppers, broccoli, carrots, celery, corn, greens, parsley, peas, pumpkin, and squash.

For men who have sperm agglutination (sperm stick together), vitamin C can help. Some experts recommend taking 1,000 mg of vitamin C daily to reduce agglutination. Foods to consider include apricots, asparagus, bell peppers, blueberries, broccoli, cabbage, cantaloupe, cauliflower, grapefruit, greens, guava, lemons, mango, onions, papaya, parsley, peaches, peas, pumpkin, strawberries, sweet potatoes, tangerines, tomatoes, and watermelon. Men who have low testosterone levels may benefit from zinc supplements, which can increase both sperm counts and fertility. In most studies, the effective dose was 25 mg three times daily for several months.

Zinc-rich foods include asparagus, calf's liver, greens, peas, pumpkin seeds, sesame seeds, and yogurt.

Vitamin B-12 is necessary to maintain fertility, and several studies support this claim. In one, infertile men took 1,500 mcg daily for four to twenty-four weeks. Sperm counts increased in fifty-four percent of men, and sperm motility increased in fifty percent. Vitamin B-12 is found in calf liver, clams, fortified cereals, fortified soy foods, salmon, tuna, and turkey. Coenzyme Q10 plays a role in sperm formation, and research shows that taking 10 mg daily for two weeks can increase sperm count and motility. The amount of CoQ10 in foods has not been well documented, but it is found in small amounts in whole grains, meats, and fish.

INSOMNIA

Do you have trouble falling asleep? Staying asleep? Do you wake up feeling tired all the time? You may have insomnia, which is defined as difficulty falling asleep, maintaining sleep, or both. An estimated thirty to fifty percent of people experience insomnia, and for ten percent of people it is a chronic condition.

Insomnia is a symptom, not a disease. It can affect people of all ages; among older adults, insomnia affects women more than men. People who have insomnia often experience problems during the day, including poor concentration, memory difficulties, irritability, and becoming drowsy or falling asleep while driving.

What Causes Insomnia?

Insomnia can have psychological or physical causes. The most common triggers of psychological-related insomnia are stress, depression, and/or anxiety. In fact, insomnia is a common symptom of depression. Physical causes of insomnia can include chronic pain, congestive heart failure, degenerative diseases (e.g., Alzheimer's disease), certain medications (e.g., those for high blood pressure), use of alcohol and/or caffeine, and menopause.

How Foods and Supplements Can Help

Did you ever wonder why your mother gave you warm milk before you went to bed? Because calcium, especially in food, has a calming effect on the body. To relieve insomnia and relax, try a glass of warm nonfat milk, some yogurt, or 600 mg of liquid calcium about forty-five minutes before you retire. Take another 600 mg of calcium after a meal earlier in the day as well. Magnesium is another mineral that can help you sleep. A suggested dose is 250 mg three to four times daily. Magnesium-rich foods include almonds, avocado, beans (dried), greens, peas, pumpkin seeds, and tofu.

The B vitamins are referred to as "stress vitamins" because they can help relieve tension. Vitamins B-5, B-6, and B-12 are especially useful for insomnia. Suggested daily doses are 100 mg of B-5, 50–100 mg of B-6, and 25 mg of B-12. Good food sources of the B vitamins are bananas, beans (dried), eggs, greens, nonfat milk, nutritional yeast, oats, peanuts, salmon, tuna, turkey, walnuts, yogurt, and whole grains.

IRRITABLE BOWEL SYNDROME

As many as twenty percent of American adults have a common disorder known as irritable bowel syndrome (IBS), yet many of them don't talk about it because they are embarrassed. Irritable bowel syndrome is characterized by abdominal bloating, gas, abdominal cramps, diarrhea, and/or constipation. Unlike diverticular disease (discussed elsewhere in this section), ulcerative colitis, or Crohn's disease, IBS does not increase your risk of colorectal cancer, nor does it cause inflammation of the intestinal tract. Many people who have irritable bowel syndrome learn to control it with diet and lifestyle changes.

What Causes Irritable Bowel Syndrome?

The exact causes of IBS are uncertain. Some experts say the symptoms are caused by changes in the nerves that control muscle contractions; others believe the central nervous system has some effect on the colon. Given that women are twice as likely as men to develop IBS, hormones may play a significant role in the disease as well.

In a healthy intestinal tract, the muscles responsible for moving food through the tract to the rectum do so in a coordinated rhythm. In people who have IBS, however, the muscle contractions may be longer than normal, resulting in diarrhea; or they may be abnormally short, causing constipation. Some people say that certain triggers set their symptoms in motion. These may include foods (e.g., chocolate, milk, carbonated beverages), stress, or medications.

How Foods and Supplements Can Help

It's useful to know which foods you should avoid and which can be beneficial if you have IBS. Generally, avoid foods that are high in fat and/or insoluble fiber—e.g., raw fruits and vegetables (but cooked is okay), red meat, dairy products, egg yolks, and fried foods—and those that can irritate the digestive tract, such as carbonated beverages, caffeine, and alcohol. Foods to enjoy include barley, brown rice, cooked fruits and vegetables, oatmeal, pasta, salmon, soy, tuna, and turkey. Beans and lentils can be eaten in moderation, as they are a good source of soluble fiber but also contain insoluble fiber.

Probiotics are proving to be beneficial for people who have IBS. Studies show improvement when patients take *Lactobacillus casei shirota*, *L. planarum*, or *E. coli nissle 1917*, although other strains may be beneficial as well. Look for a supplement that contains a variety of beneficial bacteria, and include low- or no-fat kefir and yogurt in your diet as well.

The spice turmeric also is effective. In one study, a daily supplement of turmeric for eight weeks reduced IBS symptoms by fifty percent or more in approximately two-thirds of the more than two hundred participants. You can use turmeric in cooking, but a supplement may be more effective. Andrew Weil, MD, founder and program director of the Program for Integrative Medicine at the University of Arizona, suggests taking 300 to 400 mg up to three times daily.

MACULAR DEGENERATION

Age-related macular degeneration (AMD) is a chronic eye disease in which the macula—the part of the retina that is responsible for central vision—is damaged. The degeneration of the macula causes blurry central vision or a blind spot in the center of the line of vision. Although people with AMD retain their peripheral vision, central vision loss eventually prevents or severely limits their ability to drive, read, watch TV, write, or do any type of detail work.

An estimated 1.75 million Americans have macular degeneration, and it is the leading cause of severe vision loss in people sixty-five years and older. The disease usually develops gradually, but in some people it progresses quickly in either one or both eyes. Although there is no cure for macular degeneration and damage to the macula cannot be reversed, early detection and treatment may reduce the extent of vision loss.

What Causes Macular Degeneration?

Macular degeneration occurs when the macula becomes damaged, largely due to aging. Over the years, the outer surface of the retina, called the retinal pigment epithelium (RPE), becomes thin, which triggers a breakdown in the exchange of nutrients and waste materials between the retina and the underlying layer of blood vessels. This deterioration damages the cells of the macula. The damaged cells can no longer transmit normal signals through the optic nerve to the brain, and vision becomes blurry.

Macular degeneration can be either dry or wet. Eighty-five to ninety percent of all cases of age-related macular degeneration are dry, in which the RPE deteriorates due to aging, and the waste products accumulate, interfering with vision. The wet form usually begins as dry, and then new blood vessels grow under the macula. These vessels leak blood or fluid, thus it is "wet." The wet form usually results in more serious vision loss.

Risk factors for developing macular degeneration include smoking (the single most preventable cause), obesity, family history of the disease, high blood pressure, stroke, long-term exposure to sunlight, and low levels of vitamins A, C, and E, and the mineral zinc.

How Foods and Supplements Can Help

In October 2001, the National Eye Institute released the results of AREDS (Age-Related Eye Disease Study), which looked at the effect of vitamins on age-related macular degeneration and cataracts. More than 4,700 adults (ages 55–80) who had either no AMD or some stage of the disease participated in the five-year, placebo-controlled study. Participants were given either zinc alone (80 mg; also 2 mg of copper for balance), antioxidants alone (vitamin C, 500 mg; vitamin E, 400 IU; beta-carotene, 15 mg), both zinc and antioxidants, or a placebo. For people at risk of developing advanced AMD, the combination of zinc and antioxidants reduced their risk by twenty-five percent. People without AMD or early AMD did not appear to benefit from the supplements.

The same AREDS study group, as well as other researchers, have found that the phytonutrients lutein and zeaxanthin can reduce the development of macular degeneration. Excellent sources of lutein and zeaxanthin include apricots, bell peppers, broccoli, carrots, corn, eggs (yolks), greens, lemons, oranges, peaches, pumpkin, sweet potatoes, squash, and watercress. Supplements of lutein/zeaxanthin of 6 mg daily (the amount found in ½ cup of spinach) has been associated with a reduced risk of macular degeneration.

MEMORY CHANGES

Memory change or memory loss (forgetfulness) is often associated with the normal aging process. In some cases, however, memory loss is a symptom of dementia, disease, or trauma. The difference between normal forgetfulness and dementia is that normal memory changes occur occasionally and do not interfere significantly with everyday activities, while dementia is persistent and progressive, and may affect a person's ability to do routine tasks. For example, people with normal memory changes may misplace their car keys, but people with dementia may lose the keys and also forget what they are used for.

What Causes Memory Loss?

The normal aging process often causes difficulties in attention, in learning new material, or in recalling information. However, it does not lead to significant memory loss unless disease or trauma is involved. In such cases, memory loss can be caused by Alzheimer's disease, head injury, seizures, alcoholism, stroke, drugs (e.g., barbiturates, fentanyl, benzodiazepines, halothane), brain tumors or infection, herpes encephalitis, or depression.

Memory changes occur with age because certain biological changes take place. Beginning in your twenties, you begin to lose brain cells and to produce less of certain hormones (e.g., DHEA) that the brain needs to function. Aging may also have an impact on how the brain stores information. Although aging usually does not have a significant impact on short-term memory (what you did five minutes ago) and remote memories (memories of your childhood), it can affect recent memory (e.g., what you had for breakfast this morning).

How Foods and Supplements Can Help

Your food choices can promote a better memory if they are rich in antioxidants. Research shows that antioxidants help slow oxidation, reduce inflammation, improve communication between brain cells, and make the brain less susceptible to buildup of amyloid plaque, which is associated with Alzheimer's disease. Some of these antioxidant-rich foods include almonds, apricots, asparagus, bell peppers, blueberries, broccoli, cabbage, cantaloupe, carrots, cauliflower, eggs (selenium), grapefruit, greens, guava, lemons, mango, oatmeal, onions, papaya, parsley, peaches, peas, pumpkin, strawberries, sunflower seeds, sweet potatoes, tangerines, tomatoes, watercress, watermelon, and wheat germ.

Magnesium also appears to be important for memory. A study at the Massachusetts Institute of Technology (MIT) found that magnesium helps regulate a critical brain substance that is key for learning and memory. The recommended dose is 400 mg daily.

A fifteen-year study found that 50 mg of beta-carotene daily improved memory, while another study found that healthy people ages fifty to seventy-five who took 800 mcg of folic acid daily for three years had memory test scores comparable to people nearly six years younger. Food sources of folic acid include asparagus, avocado, beans (dried), beets, bell peppers, broccoli, cabbage, cauliflower, corn, fortified cereals, greens, oranges, papaya, parsnips, peas, soybeans, tofu, turkey, and wheat germ.

If you want to spice it up a bit, a recent study found that turmeric (curcumin is the active ingredient) may help the body fight the accumulation of plaque, which is characteristic of Alzheimer's disease. As a supplement, the suggested dose of turmeric is one that provides 400 to 600 mg (three times daily) in a form standardized to curcumin content.

MENOPAUSE

Women today spend about one-third of their life in menopause, a term used to describe the changes women experience as the reproductive period of their lives gradually ends. For the majority of women, menopause evolves naturally sometime after age forty. Menopause that occurs before that time, regardless of the cause, is called premature menopause.

The process of menopause consists of three stages: perimenopause, menopause, and postmenopause. Each stage is associated with certain symptoms, although there is much overlap between the stages. The number, frequency, and severity of symptoms vary greatly among women, and for individual women as well.

What Causes Menopause?

Menopause usually begins when women are in their late thirties. That's when the ovaries, which produce and store eggs, and make the hormones that regulate menstruation and ovulation (estrogen and progesterone), start manufacturing less of the hormones. The ovaries have fewer eggs ripening each month, and ovulation becomes less regular. During their forties, periods often become more irregular, and more or less frequent. This stage of declining hormone and egg production is called perimenopause.

Once the ovaries stop releasing eggs and producing most of their estrogen, menstrual periods stop. Menopause is considered "final" when a woman has gone without a period for twelve consecutive months. Many women experience various symptoms during the latter part of perimenopause and menopause, including hot flashes, anxiety, mood swings, sleep problems, vaginal dryness, night sweats, and an urge to urinate more often. The years that follow the start of menopause are called postmenopause. The ovaries produce only a small amount of estrogen and no progesterone, and periods have ceased.

How Foods and Supplements Can Help

The ability of vitamin E to relieve hot flashes and night sweats is claimed by many women and in numerous articles, but there is little scientific evidence to back it up. However, the reported successful dose is 400 to 800 IU daily. Supplementation with calcium and magnesium can help prevent bone loss associated with the sharp decline in estrogen, and also relieve sleep difficulties. Suggested doses are 1,000 to 2,000 mg calcium and 500 to 750 mg magnesium daily. Foods that provide calcium (e.g., almonds, broccoli, greens, salmon (with bones), sesame seeds, tofu, and yogurt) and magnesium (e.g., almonds, avocado, beans (dried), greens, peas, pumpkin seeds, tofu) are recommended as well.

Probiotics can enhance how your body metabolizes and uses estrogen. A supplement that contains 1 to 2 billion CFUs of *Lactobacillus acidophilus* and several other beneficial bacteria is recommended. Include probiotic foods, such as kefir, tempeh, or yogurt in your diet as well.

NAUSEA/VOMITING AND MORNING SICKNESS

Nausea is a sensation of uneasiness of the stomach that is often accompanied by the urge to vomit, although vomiting does not always occur. Both nausea and vomiting are symptoms—not diseases—of many different conditions. Morning sickness is experienced by up to ninety percent of pregnant women during their first trimester. Its two characteristic symptoms are nausea (experienced by an estimated fifty to ninety percent of women) and vomiting (twenty-five to fifty-five percent).

What Causes Nausea/Vomiting and Morning Sickness?

Nausea and vomiting can be caused by a wide range of conditions, including infection, food poisoning, motion sickness, overeating, blocked intestinal tract, concussion, brain injury, appendicitis, migraine, brain tumors, kidney or liver disorders, heart attack, and some types of cancer. People who undergo radiation therapy or chemotherapy also often experience nausea and/or vomiting.

Morning sickness is believed to be caused by the increase in hormone levels that occurs during pregnancy, although some experts say psychological factors and evolutionary adaptation may be involved as well. The nausea, and sometimes vomiting, typically begin around the sixth week of pregnancy and lasts for about six weeks. Many health-care providers believe morning sickness is a good sign because it means the placenta is healthy.

How Foods and Supplements Can Help

If you feel nauseous, avoid foods that are fried, spicy, greasy, or sweet. Drink liquids between meals rather than with meals. Foods that may help relieve nausea or that you may be able to "keep down" include brown rice, ginger, green tea, lemons (lemonade), nonfat milk, soda crackers, watermelon, whole wheat toast (plain), and yogurt (without fruit). If you tend to feel nauseous when you get up in the morning, keep crackers by your bedside and eat them before getting out of bed. You can also eat a high-protein snack (kefir, nonfat milk, turkey, yogurt) before going to bed.

Probiotics can relieve nausea and vomiting because they help stabilize the environment in the intestinal tract. A dose of 1 to 2 billion CFUs of a probiotic supplement that contains a variety of beneficial bacteria (e.g., *Lactobacilli acidophilus*, *L. rhamnosus GG*, *L. casei*, *Bifidobacteria bifidum*, among others) is recommended.

OBESITY

Obesity and overweight are not the same. Obesity means you have too much body fat: women whose body fat (body mass index, or BMI) is greater than thirty percent of their total weight and men whose BMI is greater than twenty-five percent are obese. Overweight means you weigh more than is normal for your size and age.

According to the National Center for Health Statistics (2006), 66 percent of adults are overweight or obese (BMI > 25) and 31.4 percent are obese (BMI >30). The number of children and adolescents aged six to nineteen years who are overweight (the term "overweight" is used for both obesity and being overweight among children and adolescents) is seventeen percent. Being obese is not just about having too much fat; it also increases your risk of arthritis, diabetes, gallstones, heart disease, infertility, osteoporosis, sleep apnea, stroke, varicose veins, and some cancers.

What Causes Obesity?

The easy answer to this question is to say that it is a behavior problem—people eat more calories than their body needs—but it is more complicated than that. Other contributing factors include lack of exercise, genetics, hormone imbalance, problems with metabolism, and cultural issues. Although it is true that eating more calories than you need packs on the pounds, it is also true that people eat too many calories for different reasons. People who eat too much because they are depressed or bored are different from people who eat too much because of cultural pressure or who have a genetic tendency for slow metabolism. Therefore it is important to identify the reason(s) behind overeating so you can successfully lose weight.

How Foods and Supplements Can Help

The first step is to establish a healthful eating plan that includes fresh fruits and vegetables, whole grains, legumes, and fish, with minimal amounts of meat, dairy, sugars, and processed foods. This approach naturally includes high-fiber foods, which not only help you feel satisfied, but also may lower insulin levels. That's important because high insulin levels may increase appetite, and high-fiber foods may curb it and bring insulin levels down. Enjoy high fiber in apples, avocado, barley, beans (dried, cooked), broccoli, brown rice, carrots, figs (dried), flaxseed, grapefruit, lentils, oats, oranges, pears, peas, squash, sweet potatoes, whole grains, and 100% bran cereals.

Many claims have been made about the use of chromium to help with weight loss. Study results, however, do not support these claims.

OSTEOPOROSIS

Osteoporosis, which literally means "porous bone," is a disease characterized by a loss of bone mass and strength. As the bones weaken, the risk of fracture increases, and once one fracture occurs, the chances of suffering another one increases. Because osteoporosis usually progresses without any symptoms or pain, many people do not know they have the disease until they experience a fracture or have their bone density tested.

An estimated ten million Americans already have osteoporosis, and an additional thirty-four million are at high risk because they have low bone mass. Women are four times more likely than men to develop the disease, primarily because of the impact of estrogen loss, because women have thinner, lighter bones, and because they tend to live longer.

What Causes Osteoporosis?

Bone loses its mass and strength for various reasons. One is age: until about age thirty, bone builds up faster than it breaks down. After thirty, however, the reverse is true, and the loss of bone mass continues until a person develops osteoporosis or steps are taken to slow or stop it.

Estrogen plays a key role in the development of osteoporosis in women. Early menopause (before age forty), the lack of estrogen after menopause, or any condition that causes a lack of menstrual periods or estrogen production can cause loss of bone mass.

Other risk factors for osteoporosis include ethnicity: white and Asian women are more prone to the disease than are black and Hispanic women. Small-boned, thin women are more likely than larger-boned, heavier women to develop the disease, while a family history of the disease is a risk factor for everyone.

How Foods and Supplements Can Help

The first nutrient that comes to mind when talking about osteoporosis is calcium. If you are at risk for or have osteoporosis, the recommended dose of calcium is 1,500 to 2,000 mg daily, along with 750 to 1,000 mg magnesium. Foods to include to help you reach these daily goals include (for magnesium) almonds, avocado, beans (dried), greens, peas, pumpkin seeds, tofu; and (for calcium) broccoli, greens, nonfat milk, salmon (with bones), sesame seeds, soy (calcium fortified), tofu, and yogurt.

The importance of vitamin D in bone health has been emphasized in recent years. A supplement of 400 IU daily is important, especially for the elderly and people who do not get at least ten to fifteen minutes of sun exposure several times a week. Foods that contain vitamin D include cod liver oil, egg yolks, nonfat milk (vitamin D fortified), salmon, and sardines.

We often neglect the mineral manganese, yet it can play an important role in bone health, as many people with osteoporosis have low levels. A daily supplement of 10 to 50 mg is suggested, and you'll find a good supply in almonds, beans (dried), greens, lentils, and walnuts as well. Another neglected mineral is boron, which improves absorption of calcium and may enhance bone mineral balance. A supplement of 3 to 5 mg daily (as sodium tetrahydroborate) can be accompanied by foods rich in boron, including almonds, beans (dried), grapes, greens, prunes, and raisins.

PARKINSON'S DISEASE

Parkinson's disease is a chronic movement disorder that affects the nerve cells (neurons) in the part of the brain that controls muscle activity. In people with Parkinson's, the neurons that make a chemical called dopamine, which is necessary for muscle coordination, are damaged. The damaged cells either malfunction or die, resulting in symptoms that may include trembling of the arms, legs, hands, and face; stiffness or rigidity of the legs, arms, and torso; poor balance and coordination; and slow, hesitant movement. As the disease progresses, people often have trouble walking, chewing, swallowing, talking, and sleeping, and may develop urinary problems, depression, and dementia.

Approximately 1 to 1.5 million Americans have Parkinson's disease. Although it usually affects people age sixty and older, about fifteen percent of those with the disease are diagnosed before age fifty. Men are affected more often than women, and whites are more likely to develop the disease.

What Causes Parkinson's Disease?

No one knows why the dopamine-producing neurons in the area of the brain called the substantia nigra become damaged and die. We do know, however, that dopamine transmits messages to parts of the brain that control coordination and movement, and a decline in dopamine causes parkinsonian symptoms.

Because dopamine-producing neurons naturally decline in number as people age, some researchers believe environmental factors, such as exposure to toxins, may speed up the loss of these neurons through free-radical damage. Genetics may also play a part. An estimated fifteen to twenty-five percent of people with Parkinson's have a family history of the disease, and scientists have identified several genes that cause Parkinson's in younger patients. Parkinson's disease is likely a combination of genetic and environmental factors, although the exact combination is not yet understood.

How Foods and Supplements Can Help

People with Parkinson's disease tend to have low levels of coenzyme Q10, and studies show that supplements of this nutrient may slow progression of early-stage disease. Dosages ranging from 300 to 1,200 mg daily have been used successfully, with patients starting with a low dose and gradually increasing over time. Coenzyme Q10 is found in very small amounts in many foods, and is most prevalent in whole grains, meats, and fish.

A study from the Netherlands found that vitamin B-6 significantly reduced the risk of developing Parkinson's disease. Foods that supply vitamin B-6 include asparagus, bananas, bell peppers, cabbage, carrots, cauliflower, celery, garlic, greens, squash, tomato, tuna, turmeric, and watermelon. The suggested supplement dose is 25 to 100 mg daily.

PEPTIC ULCERS

Peptic ulcers are sores that develop on the lining of the digestive tract, including the esophagus, stomach, duodenum, and intestines. The majority of ulcers form in the duodenum (the first part of the intestinal tract) and are called duodenal ulcers; those in the stomach are called gastric ulcers.

Peptic ulcers affect more than twenty-five million Americans, and they can recur. Men and women are affected about equally.

What Causes Ulcers?

At one time, people blamed stress, coffee, and spicy foods for their ulcers. Now experts know that about ninety percent of peptic ulcers are caused by the bacteria *Helicobacter pylori*, an organism that lives and grows on the stomach lining.

The bacteria can live in the stomach for many years and not cause symptoms. It is not known exactly why some people develop ulcers from the infection and others do not.

Once an area of irritation has started to form in the digestive tract, stomach acids can contribute to ulcers by burning the lining. Physical and emotional stress can aggravate any ulcers that have developed. Other causes of peptic ulcer include alcoholism and the use of anti-inflammatory medications, including aspirin, ibuprofen, naproxen, and some prescription drugs used for arthritis.

Symptoms of peptic ulcers include a burning or gnawing pain in the abdomen, pain two to three hours after eating, heartburn, indigestion, nausea, poor appetite, belching, and pain that worsens when your stomach is empty.

How Foods and Supplements Can Help

To help prevent and treat peptic ulcers, include plenty of foods that contain flavonoids (e.g., apples, celery, cranberries, green tea, onions), which may inhibit the growth of *H. pylori*. Fiber may also reduce the risk of developing ulcers and speed your recovery as well. High-fiber foods include apples, avocado, barley, beans (dried, cooked), broccoli, brown rice, carrots, figs (dried), flaxseed, grapefruit, lentils, oats, oranges, pears, peas, squash, sweet potatoes, whole grains, and 100% bran cereals.

Probiotics, including *Lactobacillus acidophilus*, *L. rhamnosus GG*, and *L. casei*, *Bifidobacteria bifidum*, among others, can kill or slow the growth of *H. pylori*, as well as protect the lining of the digestive system against further attack. A suggested dosage for preventive purposes is 1 to 2 billion CFUs daily, of five or more species, with much higher doses recommended to treat active ulcers (e.g., 11 to 16.5 CFUs with each meal until symptoms resolve), according to John R. Taylor, ND, author of *The Wonder of Probiotics*.

The role of vitamin C in treating peptic ulcer is uncertain. In one study, high doses taken for four weeks eliminated *H. pylori* in some but not all patients. Because *H. pylori* appears to interfere with absorption of vitamin C, and low levels of vitamin

C are associated with a higher risk of stomach cancer, it is important to get enough of this nutrient. Enjoy foods like apricots, asparagus, bell peppers, blueberries, broccoli, cabbage, cantaloupe, cauliflower, grapefruit, greens, guava, lemons, mango, onions, papaya, parsley, peaches, peas, pumpkin, strawberries, sweet potatoes, tangerines, tomatoes, and watermelon to help you meet that goal; a daily supplement of 500 to 1,000 mg is also suggested.

Use of turmeric (curcumin) for peptic ulcer has a long tradition in Ayurvedic and Chinese medicine, and scientific research has shown that turmeric extract can reduce the release of stomach acid and protect against inflammation and ulcers. Studies have successfully used 750 mg to 1,500 mg of turmeric daily in three to four divided doses. Because very high levels of turmeric may induce ulcers, it is important to only take doses recommended by your health-care professional.

PREMENSTRUAL SYNDROME (PMS)

Most women who menstruate are familiar with premenstrual syndrome (PMS), a group of symptoms that occur the week or two before menstruation begins. In fact, the American College of Obstetricians and Gynecologists reports that at least eighty-five percent of menstruating women have at least one PMS symptom each month. It's been said that there are about 150 signs and symptoms of PMS, some of which include mood swings, depression, insomnia, headache, breast tenderness, joint and muscle pain, fatigue, food cravings, dizziness, nausea, diarrhea, bloating, palpitations, acne, change in sex drive, and weight gain. Most women experience mild symptoms, but up to eight percent have severe symptoms and a form of PMS called Premenstrual Dysphoric Disorder (PMDD).

Symptoms of PMS can occur in menstruating women of any age, but they occur most often in women who are in their late twenties to early forties and who have at least one child. A family history of depression and a personal past history of a mood disorder or postpartum depression is also common. The severity of symptoms can vary greatly among women, and even from month to month for the same woman.

What Causes PMS?

Experts believe that PMS is caused by a sensitivity to the hormonal changes that occur during the second half of the menstrual cycle. During the week or two before menstruation begins, estrogen and progesterone trigger changes in certain chemicals in the brain. Changes to serotonin, for example, may trigger depression and cravings for carbohydrates; fluctuations in endorphin levels may cause pain, while altered norepinephrine levels can cause mood swings. Imbalances in magnesium and calcium levels may also be a factor.

How Foods and Supplements Can Help

Researchers at the University of Massachusetts found that women who had the highest intake of calcium and vitamin D were significantly less likely to develop PMS. Suggested daily intake of calcium is 1,200 mg; of vitamin D, 400 IU. Be sure to include calcium-rich foods (broccoli, greens, nonfat milk, salmon (with bones), sesame seeds, soy [calcium fortified], tofu, and yogurt) and to get exposure to sunlight for about fifteen minutes several times per week, along with enjoying foods with vitamin D (e.g., egg yolks, nonfat milk [vitamin D fortified], salmon, and sardines).

Magnesium can help reduce PMS symptoms. In one study, women who took 250 mg of magnesium beginning twenty days after the first day of their period until the beginning of their next period experienced significantly reduced symptoms. Consider magnesium-rich foods as well: almonds, avocado, beans (dried), greens, peas, pumpkin seeds, and tofu. Take magnesium along with calcium and vitamin D for maximum effect.

Some women and health-care practitioners say taking vitamin B-6 helps relieve PMS symptoms, but scientific evidence is inconclusive. To see if you get results, take 25 to 100 mg of the vitamin beginning several days before your period starts and continue until it ends. Foods that provide good levels of vitamin B-6 include asparagus, bananas, bell peppers, cabbage, carrots, cauliflower, celery, garlic, greens, squash, tomato, tuna, turmeric, and watermelon.

PROSTATE ENLARGEMENT

For men older than fifty a common health concern is prostate enlargement, or benign prostatic hyperplasia. Symptoms rarely occur before age forty but more than fifty percent of men in their sixties and up to ninety percent of men in their seventies and eighties have some symptoms of BPH, although they may be mild. Signs and symptoms of BPH include an interrupted, weak urine stream, dribbling, leaking, urgency to urinate, and more frequent urination, especially during the night.

What Causes Prostate Enlargement?

The prostate gland continues to grow throughout a man's lifetime, but why it does so is unknown. One theory involves hormones. Men produce both testosterone (a male hormone) and a very small amount of estrogen (a female hormone). As men age, the amount of testosterone decreases, leaving a higher proportion of estrogen, which may stimulate prostate cell growth. Another idea is that dihydrotestosterone (DHT), which is derived from testosterone, may promote growth of the prostate. Most animals stop producing DHT as they age, but older men continue to manufacture it. Among men who don't make DHT, however, prostate enlargement does not occur.

As the prostate continues to enlarge, it often presses against the surrounding tissue, including the urethra, which carries urine out of the body. The pressure irritates the bladder, causing it to contract even when it does not contain much urine. This stimulates frequent urination. As the bladder becomes weaker and unable to completely empty itself, some urine remains and may cause bladder infection.

How Foods and Supplements Can Help

Studies on which nutrients may help prevent and treat BPH have yielded mixed results. One at the University of Maryland, for example, found that zinc inhibited prostate cancer cell growth in human cells. The suggested dose is 50 mg once daily; foods that provide zinc include asparagus, calf's liver, greens, peas, pumpkin seeds, sesame seeds, and yogurt.

Beta-carotene and vitamin C may offer some benefits. A large ten-year study in Italy found that beta-carotene use was associated with a significant decrease in risk of developing BPH, while vitamin C showed a lesser but still important decreased risk. A recommended dose of beta-carotene is 5,000 IU daily; for vitamin C, 500 to 1,000 mg daily. Foods that supply beta-carotene and/or vitamin C include apricots, asparagus, bell peppers, blueberries, broccoli, cabbage, cantaloupe, carrots, cauliflower, grapefruit, greens, guava, lemons, mango, oatmeal, onions, papaya, parsley, peaches, peas, pumpkin, strawberries, sweet potatoes, tangerines, tomatoes, and watermelon.

PSORIASIS

Psoriasis is a common, chronic skin condition that can strike people of all ages. The most common type of psoriasis is plaque psoriasis, in which patches of itchy or burning red plaques form anywhere on the skin, but most often on the knees, elbows, or scalp. Approximately 5.5 million people have plaque psoriasis, and about one-third of them also have psoriatic arthritis, which is characterized by joint inflammation. Plaque psoriasis occasionally evolves into a more severe form of the disease called pustular psoriasis, in which blisters containing pus form on the skin. Pustular psoriasis usually covers a wide area and it can be painful.

Psoriasis affects men and women equally. Two age groups are more susceptible to outbreaks of psoriasis: people between ages sixteen and twenty-two, and those between fifty-seven and sixty. The disease is not contagious, but it can be inherited.

What Causes Psoriasis?

Research indicates that psoriasis likely is an autoimmune disease, which means that the immune system has an abnormal reaction to healthy cells. In psoriasis, the T cells, which are a type of white blood cell that protect the body against infection, trigger skin inflammation and cause the skin cells to grow abnormally fast and accumulate in patches. Factors that may trigger an outbreak of psoriasis include smoking, alcoholism, emotional stress, hormone changes (e.g., during adolescence and menopause), HIV infection, and exposure to the sun.

Some people have genes that make them more likely to develop psoriasis. If both parents have psoriasis, any children they have are born with a fifty percent chance of developing the disease.

How Foods and Supplements Can Help

Omega-3 fatty acids can significantly improve symptoms of psoriasis, especially inflammation, according to several studies. A recommended dose of omega-3 supplement for psoriasis is 1,000 to 3,000 mg daily. Talk to your doctor about the best dose for your needs. You can help meet your goals by including omega-3–rich foods in your diet, including avocados, Brazil nuts, flaxseed, salmon, sardines, tuna, and walnuts.

Turmeric (curcumin) can reduce inflammation and fight free-radical damage associated with psoriasis. Season your vegetables, grains, soups, salads, and stews with turmeric/curcumin often. As a supplement, the suggested dose should provide 400 to 600 mg (two to three times daily) in a form standardized to curcumin content.

Although there are no firm studies on the use of probiotics for psoriasis, anecdotal reports say that the beneficial bacteria help relieve symptoms. A recommended dose is 1 to 2 billion CFUs daily of a probiotics supplement that contains three or more species, including *Lactobacilli acidophilus*, *L. ramnosus GG*, and *Bifodobacteria* sp. Also include probiotics foods, including kefir, tempeh, and yogurt in your daily diet.

Shingles

Shingles is a viral infection in which the same organism that causes chicken pox—the herpes zoster virus—is reactivated many years after it has been dormant. Once a person has had chicken pox, the virus remains inactive in the root of nerves that regulate sensation. When the virus "wakes up" decades later, it travels along a sensory nerve and causes a painful, even excruciating, rash called shingles.

About twenty percent of people who had chicken pox or the vaccine as children can expect to get shingles in adulthood. People who have a compromised immune system (e.g., cancer, HIV) are more susceptible to shingles, yet most people who get shingles are healthy. Shingles is not contagious, and it cannot cause herpes infection. A person with shingles can, however, transmit the virus to anyone who has never had chicken pox.

What Causes Shingles?

No one has identified an exact cause for reactivation of the chicken pox virus that results in shingles. Stress, fatigue, a weakened immune system, age, presence of cancer, radiation therapy, and injury to the skin where the outbreak of shingles occurs have been named as possible triggers. The rash typically develops on one side of the body only, and appears as a band of blisters from the middle of the back around the chest on one side to the breastbone. The face, neck, and scalp may be involved as well.

Along with pain, people with shingles can also experience tingling, numbness, or extreme sensitivity in certain parts of the body, fever and chills, headache, and upset stomach. Although an episode of shingles usually resolves by itself within a few weeks, prompt treatment can relieve the pain and speed up recovery.

How Foods and Supplements Can Help

A recent study published in the *International Journal of Epidemiology* found that among older people, a combination of vitamins (A, B-6, C, E, folic acid), minerals (iron, zinc), and fruit and vegetable consumption helped reduce the risk of developing shingles. Other studies show that antioxidants are helpful in managing herpes viruses. Rather than list the individual foods that include all of these nutrients, we encourage you to enjoy the items included in the "Foods" section of this book, with emphasis on the fruits and vegetables.

Along with the suggested antioxidant foods, a daily

supplement program is also recommended to help prevent and manage shingles: 5,000 IU vitamin A/beta-carotene; 25–100 mg vitamin B-6; 500–1,000 mg vitamin C; 400 IU vitamin E; 400 mcg folic acid; 15 to 30 mg zinc; 15 to 30 mg iron; and 100 to 200 mcg selenium.

Oatmeal can provide relief from itching and burning, but you don't have to eat it to get the benefits. Mix uncooked oatmeal with a small amount of water until it forms a paste, then apply the paste to the rash. Repeat as needed.

STROKE

Every forty-five seconds, someone in the United States suffers an interruption of blood flow to the brain resulting in stroke, or brain cell death. The most common type of stroke is ischemic, in which a blood clot blocks the flow of blood in a vessel in the brain. Eighty percent of strokes are this type. A hemorrhagic stroke occurs when a blood vessel breaks and leaks blood into the brain. A "ministroke" or transient ischemic attack (TIA) occurs when the blood supply to the brain is interrupted only briefly. Stroke kills more than 150,000 Americans each year, or one person every three minutes.

Do you know the symptoms of stroke? Rapid recognition and immediate medical attention can save lives. They are:

- sudden numbness or weakness of the face and/or limbs, especially on one side of the body
- sudden confusion, difficulty talking or understanding speech
- sudden dizziness, loss of balance or coordination, or difficulty walking
- sudden severe, unexplained headache
- sudden difficulty with vision

What Causes Stroke?

An ischemic stroke is most often the result of vessel damage caused by high blood pressure, diabetes, or hardening of the arteries (atherosclerosis). In other cases a blood clot or a piece of plaque from an artery wall or the heart breaks loose and clogs an artery in the brain. A hemorrhagic stroke occurs when a blood vessel in the brain ruptures and bleeds into the surrounding tissue. This usually occurs because of high blood pressure or an aneurysm—a weak spot in the blood vessel which causes it to bulge and burst.

Risk factors for stroke include high blood pressure, smoking, high cholesterol, use of birth control pills or hormone therapy, high homocysteine levels, uncontrolled stress, diabetes, certain heart problems (e.g., atrial fibrillation), and aging.

How Foods and Supplements Can Help

Coenzyme Q10 is often referred to as a heart nutrient, and one reason is that it increases blood flow to the brain. The suggested dosage is 30 to 60 mg three times daily. Omega-3 fatty acids are also heart-friendly because they fight free radicals and inflammation. Take 500 to 1,000 mg two or three times daily if you are at risk for stroke.

Vitamin C and various bioflavonoids, especially rutin, strengthen and heal blood vessel walls. A suggested dosage is 500 to 1,000 mg of vitamin C with an equal amount of mixed bioflavonoids three times daily. Foods that provide vitamin C and bioflavonoids can help you reach these goals: almonds, apricots, asparagus, bell peppers, blueberries, broccoli, cabbage, cantaloupe, carrots, cauliflower, grapefruit, greens, guava, lemons, mango, oatmeal, onions, papaya, parsley, peaches, peas, pumpkin, strawberries, sweet potatoes, tangerines, tomatoes, watercress, and watermelon.

Vitamin E may be helpful, but talk to your doctor before taking this supplement, as results are mixed. Some studies show that vitamin E reduces LDL (bad) cholesterol and increases HDL (good) cholesterol; others do not. A 2007 study in the *American Journal of Clinical Nutrition*, for example, found an improvement in LDL but not HDL levels when vitamin E was added to a high-cholesterol diet in baboons. Supplemental vitamin E may reduce the risk of blood clots, but it also may increase your risk of hemorrhagic stroke. The typical recommended dosage is 200 to 400 IU daily.

Two B vitamins associated with reduced risk of stroke are B-6 and folate, both of which help prevent high levels of a known risk factor for stroke, homocysteine. Try 300 mg of vitamin B-6 and 800 mcg of folic acid daily to help keep this risky substance under control. You can enjoy vitamin B-6 in asparagus, bananas, bell peppers, cabbage, carrots, cauliflower, celery, garlic, greens, squash, tomato, tuna, turmeric, and watermelon, and folate in asparagus, avocado, beans (dried), beets, bell peppers, broccoli, cabbage, cauliflower, corn, fortified cereals, greens, oranges, papaya, parsnips, peas, soybeans, tofu, turkey, and wheat germ.

URINARY TRACT INFECTION

Urinary tract infection (UTI) is a broad term for infections that can occur in the kidneys, bladder, ureters (the tubes that carry urine from the kidneys to the bladder), and/or the urethra (the tube that carries urine from the bladder to outside the body). Urinary tract infections usually develop first in the bladder (called cystitis) or urethra (urethritis). If the infection progresses to the kidneys and ureters, the result is a kidney infection (pyelonephritis).

Approximately eight to ten million people in the United States develop a UTI each year. The majority of cases occur in women; UTIs are ten times more common among women, and twenty percent of women can expect to experience at least one UTI. Urinary tract infections are rare in boys and young men.

What Causes Urinary Tract Infections?

The most common culprit in UTIs are the bacteria *Escherichia coli*, which normally live in the colon. (*Chlamydia* and *Mycoplasma* may also cause UTIs in women and men, but these infections rarely extend beyond the urethra and reproductive system.) Normally, urine is germ free when it leaves the body, and during urination it sweeps out any bacteria that may be in the urethra. Sometimes, however, bacteria in the urinary tract are not handled by the body's immune system and they reproduce, causing an infection. The bacteria may reach the urethra because of poor hygiene (improper wiping after using the toilet), especially because the urethral opening is very near the anus in women.

Use of a catheter also is associated with frequent urinary tract infections. A UTI can develop if the urge to urinate is often ignored, or during pregnancy, when the bladder can be compressed by the fetus, thus preventing the bladder from emptying completely and allowing bacteria to multiple. For many women, sexual intercourse triggers an infection, as can use of a diaphragm.

How Foods and Supplements Can Help

To put the brakes on a UTI when you get a hint one is developing (burning during urination is a clue), take vitamin C (500 mg twice daily) and cranberry (400 mg twice daily) to make your urine more acidic and thus less inviting for the bacteria. Foods high in vitamin C (e.g., apricots, asparagus, bell peppers, blueberries, broccoli, cabbage, cantaloupe, cauliflower, grapefruit, greens, guava, lemons, mango, onions, papaya, parsley, peaches, peas, pumpkin, strawberries, sweet potatoes, tangerines, tomatoes, watermelon) are also recommended. Cranberry, both as a supplement and the fruit and/or juice (unsweetened), also prevents the bacteria from sticking to the lining of the urinary tract.

To bolster the immune system when faced with a UTI, some experts recommend taking 25,000 to 50,000 IU daily of beta-carotene (also found in apricots, cantaloupe, carrots, greens, mango, oatmeal, papaya, peaches, peas, pumpkin, sweet potatoes, tomatoes), along with 30 mg of zinc (food sources include asparagus, calf's liver, greens, peas, pumpkin seeds, sesame seeds, and yogurt).

Finally, drinking lots of water increases urine flow and thus helps eliminate the bacteria from your system. At the first hint of an infection, or if you have a UTI, drink one eight-ounce glass of water every two hours.

VARICOSE VEINS

Varicose veins are swollen, enlarged veins that are common among people older than fifty; in fact, this condition affects half of the adults in that age group. Varicose veins can be blue to dark purple, and are usually located on the inside of the leg or backs of the calves.

For most people with varicose veins, the condition is a cosmetic issue. Symptoms can include achy or itchy legs, or legs that feel heavy, and these symptoms can worsen if you stand for long periods of time. Some people experience severe pain when standing or have cramps in their legs at night.

What Causes Varicose Veins?

The veins in the legs work very hard, against gravity, to return blood to the heart. The one-way valves in the veins allow blood to flow toward the heart and then they close to prevent blood from flowing backward. Over time, veins can become less elastic and the valves can weaken, which means some of the blood that should flow toward the heart leaks backward. The leaking blood forms tiny pools in the veins and they become twisted and inflamed. Varicose veins are blue because the blood lacks oxygen.

Several factors can contribute to the development of varicose veins. Routinely standing for extended periods of time can interfere with blood flow, as can being obese, which places additional pressure on the veins. Pregnant women often develop varicose veins because changes in blood flow that occur during pregnancy reduce the flow of blood from the legs to the pelvis.

How Foods and Supplements Can Help

A diet high in fiber (25–30 grams daily) is recommended to prevent varicose veins because it helps avoid the need to strain, which builds up pressure and irritates varicose veins. Many whole foods (e.g., apples, avocado, barley, beans (dried, cooked), broccoli, brown rice, carrots, flaxseed, grapefruit, lentils, oats, oranges, pears, peas, squash, whole grains, and 100% bran cereals) are good sources of fiber.

To strengthen vein walls and improve circulation, get plenty of vitamin C and bioflavonoids, especially rutin. Vitamin C can be found in many foods, including apricots, asparagus, bell peppers, blueberries, broccoli, cabbage, cantaloupe, cauliflower, grapefruit, greens, guava, lemons, mango, onions, papaya, parsley, peaches, peas, pumpkin, strawberries, sweet potatoes, tangerines, tomatoes, and watermelon. You can get the best of both nutrients if you focus on apricots, berries, and citrus. These fruits are a good source of rutin, which research shows can benefit varicose veins. Suggested supplement dosages are 1 to 5 g of vitamin C plus 100 to 1,000 mg bioflavonoids daily in divided doses, or take 50 mg of rutin twice daily instead of the mixed bioflavonoids.

Vitamin E improves circulation, especially in blood vessels in the legs. Before you take this potent antioxidant, however, talk to your health-care provider, especially if you are taking blood-thinning medications or if you have high blood pressure. Your doctor may start you at 200 IU daily and increase it to a level suitable for you. Include foods that provide vitamin E in your diet as well; for example, almonds, broccoli, greens, kiwi, mango, peanut butter, sunflower seeds, wheat germ oil.

VAGINITIS

Vaginitis is a broad term that refers to any infection or inflammation of the vagina. The most common types of vaginitis are yeast infections, bacterial vaginosis, atrophic vaginitis, and trichomoniasis. Each type of vaginitis is caused by a different factor, yet many of their symptoms are shared: vaginal burning and/or itching, an abnormal vaginal discharge that may be thick and/or odorous, burning when urinating, and pain during intercourse. Most women will experience at least one bout of vaginitis in their lifetime, and they may also have more than one type simultaneously.

What Causes Vaginitis?

Yeast infections are caused by any one of the fungus species called Candida, which normally live in balance in the vagina. An imbalance can occur if you take antibiotics, have diabetes, or become pregnant, and an infection takes over. An estimated seventy-five percent of women get at least one yeast infection during their life.

In bacterial vaginosis, certain bacteria grow out of control, but the cause is unknown. This type affects more than sixteen percent of pregnant women in the United States. The sharp decline in estrogen levels at menopause is the main cause of atrophic vaginitis, which results in drying and thinning of the vaginal walls. Up to forty percent of postmenopausal women get atrophic vaginitis. Trichomoniasis is a sexually transmitted infection caused by the parasite *Trichomonas vaginalis*.

How Foods and Supplements Can Help

Probiotics can launch an aggressive campaign against the bacteria that can cause certain types of vaginitis. *Lactobacillus acidophilus*, for example, acts like an antiobitic and prevents the growth of Candida and unfriendly bacteria. This bacterium can be effective if it is taken orally or applied into the vagina. If bacterial vaginosis or Candida occurs, the treatment recommended by John R. Taylor, ND, author of *The Wonder of Probiotics*, includes taking 16.5 billion CFUs of as many species as possible at each meal for five days, then gradually reducing the dose to a maintenance dose of 2 billion CFUs daily. Some of the species effective against bacterial vaginosis are *L. rhamnosus* GR-1 and *L. reuteri* RC-14; *L. acidophilus* has been effective against *Trichomonas* infection. You should also include probiotic foods in your diet every day, including fermented vegetables, kefir, tempeh, and yogurt.

Vitamin E may provide some relief if it is used as a suppository in the vagina or if the oil is applied to the vaginal area to soothe the mucous membranes. You may also try garlic, which is an antimicrobial agent. Include one to two cloves per day to help fight a yeast infection or a case of bacterial vaginosis.

PART II
Top 80+ Medicinal Foods

APPLES

Apples are one of the oldest and most popular fruits, and we can probably thank the ancient Romans for bringing them to our tables. The wild apples of ancient Asia were tiny and sour, and researchers believe the Romans found a way to cultivate larger, sweet fruits. By the first century, dozens of apple varieties were being grown; 643 different types were documented in 1866 in *Downing's Fruits*, and today there are at least 7,500 different varieties that vary in color, juiciness, sweetness, shape, nutritional value, and other characteristics.

Apple Nutrition
   Serving Size: 1 small (3 apples/lb)
   Calories: 77
   Protein: 0 g
   Total Fat: 0 g
   Carbohydrates: 20 g
   Fiber: 3.6 g
   Cholesterol: 0 mg
   Vitamin C: 7.9 mg, 9% DRI

Apples also are a good source of quercetin (a flavonoid; see "Health Benefits") as well as a fair amount of boron, iron, and vitamin B2.

Health Benefits

The secret behind the "An apple a day" adage is that this fruit has a combination of nutrients that help fight everything from cancer to constipation to heart disease. Many of those nutrients, including antioxidants, are in the skin. That means if you peel an apple, you remove about fifty percent of its antioxidant power. Let's look at the benefits of apples.

- Apples contain pectin, a soluble fiber that supports the growth of good bacteria in the digestive system, which in turn promotes healthy digestion. Pectin also reduces cholesterol levels by lowering insulin secretion.
- The high fiber content of apples helps keep you "regular" and thus avoid constipation.
- The vitamin C protects cells from damage and supports healthy blood vessels.
- Eating raw apples cleans the teeth and massages the gums, which can ward off gingivitis.
- Quercetin, a common flavonoid and antioxidant found in apple skin (but not the pulp), has anti-inflammatory properties, which helps in conditions such as arthritis and prostate enlargement.
- According to Dr. Barry Sears in *The Top 100 Zone Foods*, including apples in your diet can help control insulin levels by slowing the release of sugar into your bloodstream. This benefit is due to the presence of pectin.
- Cornell University researchers found that apple extract inhibits both colon and liver cancer cell growth. Lung cancer also seems to respond to apples. In the August 1997 issue of *American Journal of Epidemiology*, investigators found that people who ate the most flavonoid-rich foods (including apples and other fruits) had a twenty percent lower incidence of cancer. Quercetin accounted for ninety-five percent of the flavonoids consumed by the participants. Take away message: don't peel your apples (and buy organic)!

How to Select and Store

Most apple varieties are available from July through December, although a few are harvested from January through April. Buy organic apples when possible (farmers markets are a great source), and avoid any that have been waxed. Apples keep best when they are refrigerated.

Always wash apples before you cut or eat them to reduce your exposure to pesticides or bacteria. Since the skin contains important nutrients, eat apples with the skin intact unless the fruit has been waxed, in which case you should peel it.

AUTUMN APPLE SALAD

Serves 1

2 cups lettuce (Romaine, red-leaf)
4 slices (2 oz) turkey breast, skinless
½ cup apple, cut into thin wedges
⅓ cup seedless grapes
¼ cup (1 oz) shredded low-fat cheddar cheese
1 Tbs lemon juice
1 Tbs red wine vinegar

Place all ingredients except the juice and vinegar on a plate or in a salad bowl in the order listed. Mix together the juice and vinegar and pour over the salad.

BREAKFAST APPLE OATMEAL

Serves 1

½ cup diced apple
⅓ cup unsweetened apple juice
⅓ cup water
⅓ cup quick-cooking rolled oats
⅛ tsp salt (optional)

Combine apples, juice, water, and salt. Bring to a boil. Stir in oats and cook 1 minute. Cover and let stand before serving.

ALMONDS

The tear-shaped almond has been a culinary favorite since
ancient times. The Romans believed they were also fertility
charms and so threw them at newlyweds. These nuts were
originally found in the Mediterranean area, including what is
now Spain, Israel, Italy, and Greece, and they were brought to
America from Spain in the mid-1700s by the Franciscan fa-
thers. It wasn't until the twentieth century, however, that almond trees were firmly established in the US, mainly in
California but also in Arizona.

Almond Nutrition
  Serving Size: ¼ cup
  Calories: 205
  Protein: 7.6 g
  Total Fat: 18 g
  Carbohydrates: 6.6 g
  Fiber: 4 g
  Cholesterol: 0 mg
  Calcium: 92 mg, 9% DRI
  Magnesium: 76 mg, 20% DRI
  Riboflavin: 0.30 mg, 25% DRI
  Vitamin E: 9 mg, 33% DRI

Health Benefits
  Almonds are a rich source of several nutrients that can play
a significant role in the prevention and treatment of various
health concerns. For example:

  • Almonds are a good source of calcium (they have
    more of this mineral than any other nut), which can
    help in the prevention of osteoporosis.
  • Ongoing research, including work at the University of
    California-Davis, indicates that almonds may help re-
    duce the risk of colon cancer. The vitamin E, fiber, and
    antioxidant polyphenols may be the elements that pro-
    vide this protection.

- When it comes to heart disease, five large studies (Nurses Health Study, Iowa Health Study, and others) found that nut consumption is associated with a lower risk for heart disease. Eating just one ounce of almonds daily significantly reduces total and LDL cholesterol by 4% and 5%, respectively. The polyphenols in almonds help prevent the oxidation of LDL cholesterol, while the high content of healthy, monounsaturated fat also is effective in reducing cholesterol.
- The potassium in almonds provides protection against high blood pressure and atherosclerosis.
- Almonds appear to reduce post-meal increases in blood sugar levels, which is helpful for diabetics.
- Results of a study published in the *International Journal of Obesity and Related Metabolic Disorders* found that including almonds in a low-calorie diet (high in monounsaturated fats) can help overweight individuals lose weight more effectively than a low-calorie diet high in complex carbohydrates.
- Results of the Nurses' Health Study indicate that women who eat at least one ounce of nuts each week have a 25% lower risk of developing gallstones.

How to Select and Store

Choose organic, dry-roasted nuts, when possible, or almonds that are still in their shells, the form that has the longest shelf life. Do not use almonds that have dark spots or mold. When buying almonds from a bulk container, be nosy: smell the almonds and only buy nuts that smell sweet and nutty. Store almonds in an airtight container in the refrigerator, where they should keep for up to six months, or in the freezer, where they will last up to one year.

CURRY GARLICKY ALMONDS
Makes 2 cups
2 cups whole organic almonds
1 Tbs olive oil
2 tsp finely minced garlic

½ tsp garlic powder
½ tsp curry powder

Preheat the oven to 250 F. Line a baking sheet with parchment paper. Mix all the ingredients in a bowl until the nuts are well coated. Place the nut mixture on the baking sheet in a single layer and cook until the nuts begin to change color—about 20 minutes. Cool on a paper towel before serving.

ROASTED ZUCCHINI AND ALMONDS
Serves 2–3
3 small zucchini, sliced thin
2 tsp salt
2 Tbs olive oil
1 clove garlic, minced
2 Tbs green olives, chopped
¼ cup almonds, chopped
2 Tbs fresh basil, chopped

Preheat oven to 400 F. Slice zucchini lengthwise into long, thin strips and place in a bowl. Salt the zucchini and let it sit for 5 minutes. Combine all the remaining ingredients and toss lightly with the zucchini. Arrange the zucchini in a single layer on an ungreased baking sheet and bake for 20 minutes.

APRICOTS

The apricot is a small, golden-orange fruit with velvety skin and sweet flesh. A cousin of the peach, it originated in China and was eventually introduced to Europe. Apricot trees were brought to Virginia in 1720, but they didn't fare well in the climate. When apricot trees were planted in California around 1792, the trees flourished, and today more than ninety-four percent of US apricots are grown there.

Apricot Nutrition
Serving Size: 3 fruits
Calories: 51
Protein: 1.5 g
Total Fat: 0.5 g
Carbohydrates: 12 g
Fiber: 2.5 g
Cholesterol: 0 mg
Vitamin A: 2,750 IU, 105% DRI
Vitamin C: 10.5 mg, 13% DRI

Health Benefits
Apricots may be small, but they pack a powerful nutritional punch. Every juicy bite offers the following health perks.

- High levels of beta-carotene and lycopene provide protection against the damage from LDL cholesterol, a leading contributor to heart disease.
- The powerful antioxidant vitamin A promotes eye health. A study of more than fifty thousand nurses found that women who consumed the most vitamin A reduced their risk of developing cataracts by nearly forty percent.
- Apricots are a good source of fiber, which supports digestive and intestinal health, and helps avoid constipation, diverticular disease, and other gastrointestinal conditions.
- Apricots are an excellent source of the carotenoid lycopene, which is associated with a reduced risk of prostate cancer. A study showed that men who frequently ate lycopene-rich foods were eighty-two percent less likely to have prostate cancer than those who consumed the least amount.

How to Select and Store
The US apricot season is from May through August, while winter apricots are typically imported from South America. Look for fruits that have a rich orange color and that are

slightly soft. Do not buy fruit that is pale or greenish. To ripen apricots, place them in a brown bag with an apple or banana, and do not refrigerate. Ripe apricots should be refrigerated.

APRICOT SALSA
Serves 6
1 lb apricots, chopped
1–2 Tbs chopped cilantro
½ tsp white wine vinegar
¼ tsp grated lime peel
2 Tbs chopped red onion
½ Tbs olive oil
½ Tbs lime juice
½ tsp minced jalapeno pepper
¼ tsp cumin

Combine all ingredients in a bowl and mix well. Chill before serving.

APPY APRICOTS
Makes 24 appetizers
12 apricots, halved and pitted
4 oz low-fat cream cheese
½ cup almonds, chopped

Soften the cream cheese and stir in the chopped almonds. Spoon the mixture into each apricot half.

ASPARAGUS

Asparagus may well break a speed record: under ideal conditions, the green stalky vegetable can grow up to ten inches in just twenty-four hours. This member of the lily family has been enjoyed since ancient times, both for its taste and for its reported ability to treat various ailments, including arthritis, infertility, and toothaches. One thing is for sure: asparagus is a powerhouse of nutrients.

When asparagus was first introduced to the United States, it was grown in New England. Today the state with the largest asparagus production is California.

Asparagus Nutrition

Serving Size: 1 cup, cooked, fresh
Calories: 43
Protein: 4.7 g
Total Fat: 0.5 g
Carbohydrates: 7.6 g
Fiber: 2.9 g
Cholesterol: 0 mg
Folate: 263 mcg; 66% DRI
Riboflavin: 0.2 mg, 17% DRI
Thiamin: 0.2 mg, 17% DRI
Vitamin A: 970 IU, 37% DRI
Vitamin C: 19 mg, 23% DRI

Health Benefits

The health benefits attributed to asparagus by our ancestors have some scientific basis. Here's what we know:

- Folate (along with vitamins B-6 and B-12) is essential for a healthy cardiovascular system, and asparagus is an excellent source of this nutrient. When folate levels are low, homocysteine (a substance that promotes atherosclerosis) levels rise, which increases the risk for heart disease. Just one cup of asparagus provides two-thirds of the daily recommended intake of folate.
- Folate is necessary to prevent birth defects. Inadequate folate during pregnancy has been linked to various birth defects, including spinal bifida.
- Asparagus is a very good source of potassium and is low in sodium, a combination that provides a diuretic effect. Thus it can help relieve ailments that involve swelling, such as arthritis and water retention associated with premenstrual syndrome (PMS).

- Asparagus contains inulin, a type of carbohydrate that is favored by the good bacteria in the intestinal tract. When good bacteria thrive, they make it very difficult for unfriendly bacteria to establish themselves in the intestinal tract and cause disease.
- Asparagus contains more glutathione, a potent anticarcinogen and antioxidant, than other vegetables and fruits analyzed to date. Glutathione supports the immune system, participates in the repair of damaged DNA, and binds to carcinogens to assist in removing them via feces and urine.

How To Select and Store

Shop for firm, fresh spears that have closed, compact tips. Contrary to popular opinion, thick stalks can be just as tender as thin ones. To store asparagus, trim the stem ends about one-quarter inch and place in moisture-proof wrapping or stand upright in two inches of cold water. Refrigerate and use within two or three days, as asparagus loses its nutritional potency quickly.

ASPARAGUS SALAD
Serves 4
1 lb asparagus, trimmed
1 tsp salt
1½ Tbs virgin olive oil
½ cup fresh mushrooms, sliced
1 tsp fresh thyme, chopped, or ½ tsp dried
½ tsp ground cumin

In a large skillet, bring 2 inches of water to a boil with the salt. Prepare a bowl of ice water and set aside. Add asparagus to the boiling water and cook 4 to 5 minutes or until barely tender. Using tongs, remove the stalks and place in the ice water for 5 minutes. Drain and set aside. In the same skillet, heat the olive oil and sauté the mushrooms, thyme, cumin, and asparagus for 3 to 4 minutes. Serve warm or chilled.

ZESTY ASPARAGUS
Serves 4
2 lb asparagus cut into 1½ inch pieces
4 tsp soy sauce
1 tsp honey
2 tsp sesame oil
2 Tbs toasted sesame seeds

Place the cut asparagus into boiling salted water and cook until tender. Drain immediately and rinse with cold water to stop the cooking process. Pat dry. Combine the remaining ingredients and pour over the asparagus. Serve warm or chilled.

AVOCADO

They are often called butter pears or alligator pears, but avocados (from the Aztec "ahuacatl") resemble a pear in shape only. The buttery smooth texture and high (healthy) fat content of this fruit are unique among fruits. This native of Central and South America has been cultivated since about 8000 BC. It was introduced to the United States in the twentieth century, where it is grown in California and Florida. California avocados (Hass is the most popular) are small, rough skinned, and have a buttery, nutty taste. Florida varieties are larger and have a smooth, bright green skin and a mild taste.

Avocado Nutrition
Serving Size: 1 cup slices
Calories: 235
Protein: 3 g
Total Fat: 22 g
Carbohydrates: 11 g
Fiber: 7 g
Cholesterol: 0 mg
Folate: 90 mcg, 23% DRI
Vitamin A: 893 IU, 34% DRI

Vitamin B-6: 0.41 mg, 27% DRI
Vitamin C: 11.5 mg, 14% DRI

Health Benefits

Some people avoid avocados because of their high fat content, but most of it is healthy, monounsaturated fat. Benefits of this fat and other nutrients in avocados include the following:

- Avocados have a positive effect on cholesterol: studies show an average seventeen percent decline in total cholesterol among people who ate avocado daily. The improvement included a drop in LDL cholesterol and triglycerides, and an increase in HDL cholesterol, all of which greatly benefit the heart.
- A significant amount of the carotenoid lutein, which is important in maintaining healthy vision, is found in avocados.
- Avocados are rich in beta-sitosterol, a natural substance that significantly lowers cholesterol.

How to Select and Store

About ninety percent of the avocados grown in the United States come from California. Florida avocados have twenty to twenty-five percent less fat and fewer calories than their West Coast relatives. However, they are less creamy and more perishable.

Select fruit that is unblemished and heavy for its size. Avocados ripen at room temperature, usually in three to five days. Ripening can be hastened if you place the fruit in a brown paper bag with an apple and store at room temperature. The fruit is ripe when it responds to gentle pressure. If your finger leaves a dent, the fruit is overripe. Do not refrigerate unripe avocados because they will not ripen properly.

GUACAMOLE

Makes 4–6 servings
3 Hass avocados, peeled and mashed
1 tomato, chopped

2 Tbs finely chopped onion
⅛ tsp garlic powder
2 Tbs lemon juice
1 Tbs chopped green chili peppers (optional)
1 tsp salt
¼ tsp pepper
1 tsp ground coriander

Combine all ingredients and mix well. Chill before serving.

BROWN RICE AND AVOCADO SALAD
Serves 4
2 cups cooked brown rice
2 cups oranges, peeled and diced
¼ cup fresh squeezed orange juice
¼ cup unsalted pumpkin seeds, toasted
1 Hass avocado, peeled and cut into ½-inch pieces
⅛ tsp dried chipotle powder
¼ tsp salt
4 large lettuce leaves (lettuce cups)

In a large bowl, combine the cooked rice, oranges, orange juice, pumpkin seeds, salt, and chipotle. Gently mix in the avocado. Add more salt if desired. Place the mixture onto lettuce leaves.

BANANAS

Bananas are believed to have first appeared in Malaysia around 4,000 years ago, after which they spread to India, Africa, and parts of Europe. Portuguese explorers introduced bananas to the Americas in 1482. Today, the main banana producing countries include Brazil, Costa Rica, Ecuador, and Mexico, all of which export the yellow fruit to the United States.

Banana Nutrition
Serving Size: 1 medium
Calories: 108

Protein: 1.2 g
Total Fat: 0.5 g
Carbohydrates: 27.6 g
Fiber: 2.8 g
Cholesterol: 0 mg
Vitamin B-6: 0.68 mg, 45% DRI
Vitamin C: 10.7 mg, 13% DRI
Potassium: 467 mg, 10% AI (Adequate Intake)

Health Benefits

Perhaps the most well-known health fact about bananas is that they are an excellent source of potassium and are low in sodium, a combination that is important in preventing and treating high blood pressure. We talk about this health benefit, as well as others, below.

- Studies show that a diet containing potassium-rich foods such as bananas lowers blood pressure and also reduces the risk of stroke.
- Potassium supports bone health by counteracting the loss of calcium associated with a high-salt diet, which most American follow.
- Eating high-fiber foods (21 grams per day), such as bananas, reduces the risk of coronary heart disease and cardiovascular disease by twelve percent and eleven percent, respectively, according to a study in *Archives of Internal Medicine*.
- Bananas can help fight ulcers in two ways: elements in bananas promote formation of a thicker protective barrier against stomach acids, and protease inhibitors in bananas help destroy ulcer-causing bacteria in the stomach.
- Bananas are an excellent source of fructooligosaccharide, a compound that supports beneficial bacteria in the colon, which in turn increases the body's ability to absorb calcium and reduces the risk of colon cancer.

- The *International Journal of Cancer* indicates that women who eat bananas four to six times per week have a fifty percent less risk of developing kidney disease than women who don't eat bananas.
- Bananas are a rich source of serotonin and norepinephrine, two substances that can help fight depression.

How to Select and Store

Bananas are available year round. Choose bananas based on when you want to use them: those with more green take longer to ripen than those that are more yellow and/or have brown spots. Choose firm, bright, and unbruised fruit with intact stems and tips. Ripen bananas at room temperature; do not refrigerate unripe bananas because this interrupts the ripening process. To hasten ripening, place bananas in a paper bag or wrap them in newspaper along with an apple, and leave them at room temperature. Ripe bananas can be refrigerated to lengthen their life, but they should be consumed within two to three days.

BANANA SMOOTHIE
Serves 1
½ cup nonfat plain yogurt
1 ripe banana
4 fresh strawberries
10 ice cubes

Place all ingredients in a blender or food processor and process until smooth.

BANANA DIP
Makes 1½ cups
1 cup ripe banana, mashed
1 tsp lemon juice
1 tsp vanilla extract
1½ tsp ground cinnamon
¼ tsp ground nutmeg
½ cup quick oatmeal, uncooked

Combine the bananas and lemon juice and blend well. Add all
the other ingredients and blend well. Use as a dip for fruit slices
(apples, pears, oranges), crackers, or dried fruit.

BARLEY

It's nutty and chewy and a great source of fiber and other essential nutrients. It's barley, a versatile cereal grain that originated in Ethiopia and Southeast Asia more than 10,000 years
ago. Barley has long been used as both a food and beverage;
in fact, a recipe for barley wine dated 2800 BC has been
found. The Spanish introduced barley to South America, and
the English and Dutch brought it to the United States in the
17th century. Today, major barley producers are Canada, the
United States, Russia, and Germany.

Barley Nutrition
  Serving Size: 1 cup pearled, cooked
  Calories: 193
  Protein: 3.5 g
  Total Fat: 0.6 g
  Carbohydrates: 44 g
  Fiber: 6 g
  Cholesterol: 0 mg
  Manganese: 0.41 mg, 21% AI
  Niacin: 3.2 mg, 21% DRI
  Selenium: 13.5 mcg, 25% DRI
  Thiamin: 0.13 mg, 11% DRI

Note: Whole-grain barley, which has only the outermost hull
removed, has approximately double the amount of fiber and
protein of pearled barley. It also has more calories (270 per
cup), and more calcium and phosphorus (not shown here).
Whole-grain barley is usually available at health food or specialty stores.

Health Benefits

Don't let the mundane look of barley fool you: it's a powerhouse of health benefits. Here's a rundown.

- Barley's high fiber content not only increases fecal transit time and thus helps prevent constipation, hemorrhoids, and colon cancer, it also provides food for the beneficial bacteria in the large intestine that are essential for maintaining a healthy colon and for overall health as well.
- The fiber in barley produces propionic acid, which helps lower cholesterol levels.
- The fiber in barley is high in beta-glucan, a substance that helps lower cholesterol by removing it via the feces.
- Barley is more effective than oats in reducing insulin and glucose response, which is good news for type 2 diabetics.
- Eating barley can help prevent gallstones. A review of nearly seventy thousand women in the Nurses Health Study found that those who ate the most fiber had a thirteen percent lower risk of developing gallstones compared with women who ate the fewest fiber-rich foods.
- The UK Women's Cohort Study (35,972 participants) found that a diet rich in fiber from whole grains (e.g., barley) provides significant protection against breast cancer among premenopausal women.
- The significant amount of copper in barley can help reduce the symptoms of rheumatoid arthritis, as this mineral works with essential enzymes to destroy free radicals and support bones, joints, and blood vessels.

How to Select and Store

Barley comes in several forms (pearled, hulled, flaked), but pearled is the most common and popular. If you buy barley from bulk containers, be sure there is no evidence of moisture. Bulk or packaged barley should be stored in a tightly covered glass container and kept in a cool, dry place (e.g., the refrigerator, especially in hot weather).

BARLEY AND TURKEY SALAD
Serves 4
2 cups cooked pearl barley (see directions)
1½ cups cooked turkey, cubed
1 can water chestnuts, drained
½ cup sliced celery
¼ cup sliced green onion
1 cup sliced fresh strawberries
Olive oil and red wine vinegar to taste

To cook barley, bring 1½ cups water to a boil. Add ½ cup un-cooked pearl barley and return to boil. Reduce heat to low, cover and cook 45 minutes or until liquid is absorbed. Cool. To make salad: combine the cooked barley, turkey, water chestnuts, celery, and onions. Drizzle olive oil and vinegar over the mixture and toss. Chill. Top with sliced strawberries when ready to serve.

BARLEY PILAF
Serves 4
½ cup sliced button mushrooms
2 tsp olive oil
1 cup pearl barley
3 cups vegetable broth
2 Tbs chopped green onion
2 Tbs grated low-fat cheese (your choice)

Heat olive oil in saucepan, add mushrooms and sauté until limp. Add barley, broth, and onion. Bring to a boil, reduce heat to low, cover, and cook 45 minutes or until liquid is absorbed. Sprinkle with cheese and serve.

BEANS

If someone says you're full of beans, take it as a compliment, because you have good taste. Beans are one of the most nutritious foods available. Beans are a major part of the diet throughout South America and Mexico, where they have flourished for more than 7,000 years. Dried beans (e.g., pinto, navy, pink, black, kidney), like lentils and peas, are legumes, and they are warehouses of nutrients, offering a rich source of protein, fiber, and carbohydrates while being very low in fat and sugar.

Bean Nutrition
Serving Size for All: ½ cup cooked

Black Beans
Calories: 114
Protein: 8 g
Total Fat: 0.5 g
Carbohydrates: 20 g
Fiber: 7.5 g
Cholesterol: 0 mg
Folate: 128 mcg, 32% DRI
Magnesium: 60 mg, 16% DRI

Navy Beans
Calories: 127
Protein: 7.5 g
Total Fat: 0.5 g
Carbohydrates: 23 g
Fiber: 9.5 g
Cholesterol: 0 mg
Folate: 127 mcg, 32% DRI
Magnesium: 48 mg, 13% DRI
Iron: 2.2 mg, 17% DRI

Kidney Beans
Calories: 124
Protein: 7.5 g
Total Fat: 0.5 g
Carbohydrates: 20 g
Fiber: 5.5 g
Cholesterol: 0 mg
Folate: 115 mcg, 28% DRI

Manganese: 0.42 mg, 21% DRI
Iron: 2.6 mg, 20% DRI
Molybdenum: 67 mcg, 149% DRI

Health Benefits

Whether you buy dried beans and cook them yourself or choose canned beans, the nutritional value is similar. If you use canned beans, choose no-salt or low-salt varieties, or rinse them in a colander before using.

- The US Dietary Guidelines 2005 recommend that all Americans eat three cups of beans per week, as beans are instrumental in reducing the risk of heart disease and some cancers, helping with weight management, and promoting regularity.
- The soluble fiber in beans helps reduce LDL levels, which in turn lowers the risk of heart disease.
- People with diabetes can benefit from beans, as the soluble fiber slows the absorption of carbohydrates and thus helps regulate blood glucose levels.
- The insoluble fiber in beans helps prevent constipation and other intestinal ailments.
- Kidney beans are an excellent source of molybdenum, which detoxifies sulfites, a preservative often found in delicatessen foods and salad bars. People who are sensitive to sulfites can experience headache, disorientation, and rapid heartbeat if they consume sulfites and their molybdenum levels are low.

NOTE: Kidney and navy beans contain high levels of purine, a substance which, if consumed in very high amounts, can cause gout or kidney stones. However, the purine in meat and fish provide a much greater risk of these health problems than the purine in beans. You would need to eat ten times the recommended daily intake (3.5 oz) of beans each day to be at greater risk of gout.

How to Select and Store

Dried beans can be purchased already packaged or loose in bulk. Once a package has been opened or if the beans are already loose, store them in a tightly closed glass jar and keep in a cool, dark place. Beans stored in this way will keep for one year or longer.

THREE-BEAN CASSEROLE
Serves 8
1 can (16-oz) each: black, navy, and kidney beans, drained
1 lb chicken breast, cut into 1-inch pieces
1 15-oz can tomato sauce
1½ cups thinly sliced carrots
2 small onions, sliced thin
½ cup vegetable broth
2 Tbs fresh thyme leaves
2 cloves garlic, chopped fine

Heat oven to 375° F. Mix all ingredients in an ungreased 3-quart casserole. Cover and bake 1 hour or until bubbly and carrots are tender.

BEAN AND RICE SOUP
Serves 6
2 cups cooked kidney or navy beans, drained
1 cup cooked long-grain rice
2 Tbs lemon juice
4 Tbs minced fresh dill (or 1 Tbs dry dill)
Pepper to taste

Place beans, rice, lemon juice, and 2 cups water in a large saucepan and bring to a boil. Cover and lower heat, simmer for 20 minutes. Stir in dill and season with pepper.

BEETS

Although the bulb, or root, of the beet plant is what most people think about when beets are mentioned, this plant was originally grown only for its leaves, which are very nutritious. The roots come in colors ranging from deep crimson to white or golden, and one variety that has alternating red and white rings. Beets can be as small as walnuts or as large as baseballs, with the smaller bulbs being more tender than the larger ones. The peak months for beets are June through October.

Beet Nutrition
Serving Size: ½ cup
Calories: 37
Protein: 1.5 g
Total Fat: 0 g
Carbohydrates: 8.5 g
Fiber: 1.9 g
Cholesterol: 0 mg
Folate: 68 mcg, 17% DRI

Health Benefits
We discuss the benefits of the bulb or root of beets here, as they differ from those of the green tops (see "Greens"). The bulbs are known primarily for their folate and fiber content, as well as various phytonutrients.

- Beets contain the phytonutrient biochanin-A, which has cancer-fighting properties.
- The folate in beets is helpful for people with anemia, atherosclerosis, depression, diarrhea, gingivitis, or osteoporosis.
- The red pigment in beets, betacyanin, is related to anthocyanin, a potent antioxidant, which may help lower blood pressure.
- The folate, vitamin C, and beta-carotene in beets can help lower homocysteine levels. High homocysteine levels are a risk factor for heart disease.

• Eating beets can help dilute bile and allow it to flow more freely, which in turn reduces the risk of gallstone formation.

How To Select and Store

Look for beets that have fresh, bright green tops attached. (Enjoy the greens as well; see "Greens".) The bulbs should be firm and heavy, not wrinkled or sprouting, nor have scales around the top surface. Before storing fresh beets, cut off the greens and leave at least one inch of the stem attached to reduce moisture loss from the roots. Store the unwashed roots in a plastic bag in the refrigerator, where they should keep for a week or longer; store the greens in a plastic bag, refrigerate, and use within a few days as they spoil quickly.

BEETCAKE
Serves 4
2 lb beets, scrubbed, peeled, and grated
1–2 tsp olive oil
2 tsp fresh rosemary, chopped coarsely
½ cup whole wheat flour
2 tsp minced garlic
¼ tsp black pepper
½ tsp salt

Place olive oil in a 12-inch skillet and preheat while preparing the beet mixture. In a bowl, place all the remaining ingredients and mix well, until the beets are well coated with flour. Press the mixture into the skillet in a pancake shape. Cook over medium heat for 8 to 10 minutes, shaking the skillet occasionally to prevent sticking. Flip the beetcake and cook on the other side for 8 to 10 minutes. Serve hot.

BEET AND SWEET SALAD
Serves 4
3 small sweet potatoes
3 beets
6 Tbs white distilled vinegar

4 Tbs olive oil
4 tsp ground coriander

Cook the beets and potatoes in separate pots—either steam or
boil—until tender. Cool, peel, and slice into thin rounds.
Whisk vinegar, oil, and coriander in a bowl. Season with salt
and pepper to taste. Add the vegetables and toss until coated.
Chill about 2 hours before serving.

BELL PEPPERS

Bell peppers, like their relatives the chili peppers, originated in
South America around 5000 BC. The seeds made their way
around the world in the hands of explorers, and this highly
adaptable vegetable plant took hold in many different climates.
Bell peppers come in an impressive array of colors: deep
green, yellow, orange, and red—all bursting with vitamins and
antioxidants. The main producers of these colorful vegetables
are Mexico, Turkey, Romania, Spain, and China.

Bell Pepper Nutrition
Serving Size for Both: 1 cup chopped, raw

Green
Calories: 30
Protein: 1g
Total Fat: 0g
Carbohydrates: 7 g
Fiber: 2.5 g
Cholesterol: 0 mg
Vitamin A: 551 IU, 21% DRI
Vitamin C: 119 mg, 145% DRI
Vitamin B-6: 0.3 mcg, 20% DRI

Red
Calories: 39
Protein: 1.5 g

Total Fat: 0 g
Carbohydrates: 9 g
Fiber: 3 g
Cholesterol: 0 g
Vitamin A: 5244 IU, 200% DRI
Vitamin C: 190 mg, 231% DRI
Iron: 0.64 mg, 5% DRI
Vitamin B-6: 0.23 mg, 15% DRI
Niacin: 1.5 mg, 10% DRI
Folate: 20 mcg, 5% DRI

Health Benefits

Although all bell peppers have impressive nutritional values, green peppers offer somewhat less value while red ones provide the most. If you grow your own peppers, leave the green ones on the vine until they ripen fully to red, and that way you reap an especially nutritious harvest!

- Red bell peppers contain the phytonutrients beta-carotene and beta-cryptoxanthin, which reduce the risk of some cancers.
- The abundance of lycopene in red bell peppers may help promote heart health and reduce the risk of prostate, cervical, and ovarian cancer.
- Beta-carotene helps fight acne and eczema, and supports eye health, helping to prevent cataracts, macular degeneration, and other vision problems.
- Bell peppers—especially red varieties—are excellent sources of vitamins A and C, two powerful antioxidants that strengthen the immune system, may reduce occurrences of infections like the common cold, and help fight more serious conditions such as heart disease and cancer.
- Red bell peppers are especially good sources of several B vitamins, including niacin, B-6, folate, and thiamin, all of which benefit people with depression and stress-related conditions.

How to Select and Store

Choose peppers that are firm, heavy for their size, have taut skin, and are free of soft spots or darkened areas. The stems should be fresh looking. Store unwashed peppers in the vegetable compartment of the refrigerator, where they should keep for up to one week.

BELL PEPPERS AND SPINACH
Serves 4

1 medium onion, chopped
1 medium green bell pepper, chopped
1 medium red bell pepper, chopped
1 Tbs olive oil
1 medium tomato, chopped
½ lb fresh spinach
¾ tsp salt
¼ tsp black pepper
¼ cup organic peanut butter

In a large saucepan, cook and stir the onion and peppers in oil until the onion is tender. Add the tomato and spinach. Cover and simmer until the spinach is tender. Add salt, pepper, and peanut butter and heat until hot.

THREE PEPPER SALAD
Serves 6 to 8

1 red bell pepper, cored and seeded
1 yellow bell pepper, cored and seeded
1 green bell pepper, cored and seeded
1 small sweet onion, peeled
¼ cup chopped fresh basil or parsley
1 Tbs rice vinegar
1 Tbs sesame oil
Salt and coarse pepper to taste
¼ cup crumbled low-fat feta cheese

Slice the peppers and onion into matchstick pieces and place in a large bowl. Add the basil or parsley, sprinkle with salt and pepper, and add rice vinegar and sesame oil, stirring well. Cover and refrigerate for about 1 hour before serving. Sprinkle with crumbled feta cheese before serving.

BLUEBERRIES

Blueberries have always grown in the wild, and they were not cultivated until the twentieth century. The Native Americans had many uses for blueberries, both as food and medicine, but the berries didn't catch on with the colonists until the Civil War, when the fruits were canned and sent to soldiers. Today, we know that in addition to being delicious and easy to eat, blueberries are one of the best sources of antioxidants among all fruits and vegetables.

Blueberry Nutrition
Serving Size: 1 cup fresh
Calories: 84
Protein: 1 g
Total Fat: 0.5 g
Carbohydrates: 21 g
Fiber: 3.6 g
Cholesterol: 0 mg
Vitamin C: 14.4 mg, 18% DRI

Note: Nutritional information is based on USDA figures. Some sources give much higher values for vitamin C. The vitamin C content of blueberries varies widely, depending on the species and growing conditions. The 14.4 mg value is generally accepted as the norm.

Health Benefits
Although blueberries have a fair amount of vitamin C, their real power is in their high phytonutrient content. Blueberries are such a rich source of phytonutrients that they provide an enormous amount of antioxidant protection. Here are some examples of why blueberries are a wise choice.

- Studies by the US Department of Agriculture indicate that the antioxidant pterostilbene, found in blueberries, is effective in reducing cholesterol.
- The antioxidants and other phytochemicals in blueberries have the ability to reduce age-associated lipid (fat) peroxidation, a process that contributes to cardiovascular disease.
- The pterostilbene in blueberries has been shown to suppress the growth of cancer cells.
- Blueberries are a good source of ellagic acid, and research shows that people who eat foods high in this phytonutrient are three times less likely to develop cancer when compared to people who consume little or no ellagic acid.
- The antioxidants in blueberries are believed to reduce the risk of urinary tract infections.

How to Select and Store
Fresh blueberries are available from May through October. Look for firm fruits that "bounce" when you shake the container. Blueberries should also have a silver-gray "bloom," which protects the skin. Discard any soft or moldy blueberries and blot the remaining berries with a paper towel before refrigerating them. Never wash blueberries until you are ready to eat them.

BLUE MOONIE
Serves 1
2 cups frozen blueberries
6–8 ice cubes (depends on desired thickness)
2 cups pineapple juice, unsweetened
1 banana

Blend all ingredients in a blender or food processor.

BLUE CARROT SALAD
Serves 6
½ tsp salt

1 cup diced red pepper
1½ cups frozen blueberries
5 medium carrots
⅓ cup walnut pieces
½ cup pineapple pieces
Juice of 1 lemon
2 tsp olive oil

Mix lemon juice, salt, pepper, and oil. Add the blueberries and let them marinate. Peel the carrots and cut into very thin slices or matchsticks. Mix the carrots, walnuts and pineapple and add to the blueberry mixture, and toss gently.

BROCCOLI

Broccoli has been called the "Crown Jewel of Nutrition," and for good reason: it has high levels of fiber, vitamins, and phytonutrients, and is very low in calories. This relative of cabbage is believed to have gotten its name from the ancient Romans, who thought the vegetable looked like miniature trees. The name "broccoli" comes from the Latin "brachium," which means branch. It's been said that the Roman emperor Tiberius had a son, Drusius, who loved broccoli so much he ate it until his urine turned green.

Records of broccoli after ancient times were virtually nonexistent until the sixteenth century, when the vegetable was grown in Italy and France. Today, ninety percent of the broccoli consumed in the United States is grown in California.

Broccoli Nutrition
Serving Size: ½ cup chopped, cooked
Calories: 27
Protein: 2 g
Total Fat: 0 g
Carbohydrates: 5.5 g
Fiber: 2.6 g
Cholesterol: 0 mg

Vitamin A: 1207 IU, 46% DRI
Vitamin C: 50 mg, 61% DRI
Calcium: 31 mg, 3% DRI
Folate: 84 mcg, 21% DRI

Health Benefits

Ounce for ounce, boiled broccoli has more vitamin C than an orange and is a great source of folate, fiber, and vitamin A. These healthful facts are just the beginning of broccoli's benefits.

- The beta-carotene and vitamin C in broccoli may help reduce the risk of cataracts, heart disease, and several types of cancer, including breast and lung cancer.
- Broccoli contains a healthy balance of insoluble and soluble fiber, which not only helps ward off constipation and diarrhea, but also has a role in preventing colon cancer, diverticulosis, and other intestinal ailments.
- A chemical called sulforaphane found in broccoli can kill the bacterium *Helicobacter pylori,* which causes ulcers.
- Sulforaphane appears to be effective against ovarian cancer.
- The phytonutrients indoles and isothiocyanates found in broccoli help stop cancer-causing agents in the body.
- The phytonutrient kaempferol in broccoli has been found to reduce the risk of coronary heart disease in women.

How to Select and Store

Peak season for broccoli is October through April, but you can get it year-round. Look for crowns that are dark green or purplish-green with tightly closed buds. The cut ends of the stalks should be closed; open ones tend to be tough and woody. Place broccoli in a plastic bag and refrigerate as soon as possible. Although it will keep for about a week, it is best to use broccoli within three days of purchase.

BROCCOLI-BEAN SOUP
Serves 6
1 Tbs olive oil
1 cup chopped onion
2 cloves garlic, chopped
4 cups broccoli, chopped
2½ cups vegetable broth
1 potato, diced
1 cup canned navy beans, drained
1 cup nonfat milk or soymilk
¼ tsp each salt and pepper

In a heavy saucepan, heat oil over medium heat and cook the onion and garlic for about 3 minutes. Add broccoli, broth, potato, and beans. Bring to a boil and reduce heat. Simmer, covered, for about 20 minutes or until vegetables are soft. In a blender or food processor, puree ½ of the vegetable mixture. Add the pureed vegetables back in the saucepan, add the milk, salt, and pepper, and stir well until heated.

BROCCOLI SALAD
Serves 4
¾ lb broccoli florets, cooked
¾ lb zucchini, raw, cut into ¼ inch slices
⅓ cup fat-free Dijon dressing
1 red bell pepper, raw, seeded and cut into strips

Steam the broccoli in a steamer basket for about 3 minutes. Transfer broccoli into a bowl, add the zucchini, bell pepper, and dressing and toss well.

BROWN RICE

Brown rice is rice in its natural "coat": white rice that has not had the bran layer removed. This means brown rice has more nutrients than processed, white rice. Archaeologists have found evidence of rice seeds dating back about 9,000 years.

Rice is a native of Asia, and travelers from other countries gradually spread it around the globe: the Arabs brought it into ancient Greece, the Moors carried it into Spain in the eighth century, and rice was introduced into South America in the seventeenth century by the Spanish. Today most of the world's rice is grown in China, Thailand, and Vietnam.

Brown Rice Nutrition

Serving Size: 1 cup cooked long-grain
Calories: 216
Protein: 5 g
Total Fat: 2 g
Carbohydrates: 45 g
Fiber: 3.5 g
Cholesterol: 0 mg
Manganese: 2.1 mg, 105% DRI
Niacin: 3 mg, 20% DRI
Selenium: 19 mcg, 34% DRI
Thiamin: 0.19 mg, 16% DRI
Zinc: 1.2 mg, 13% DRI

Health Benefits

Brown rice is nutritionally superior to white rice in nearly every way because the process used to produce white rice robs the grain of its nutrients. The complete milling and polishing that transforms brown rice into white rice destroys about one-third of its vitamin B-3 and iron, half of its manganese and phosphorus, eighty percent of vitamin B-1, ninety percent of vitamin B-6, and all of the fiber, along with other nutrients. By law in the United States, makers of white rice must enrich their product with vitamins B-1 and B-3, and iron, but about one dozen other nutrients are not replaced. Your best bet: choose brown rice.

• Selenium works with glutathione peroxidase to help ward off cancer, and it is a powerful antioxidant that helps prevent heart disease and relieve symptoms of asthma and rheumatoid arthritis.

- Manganese assists in producing energy from protein and carbohydrates, which helps fight fatigue and to maintain a healthy nervous system.
- Brown rice contains the phytonutrients called lignans, some of which are transformed in the intestines into enterolactone, a substance believed to protect against heart disease and hormone-dependent cancers like breast cancer.
- Magnesium can help reduce the risk of type 2 diabetes because it works with enzymes that help the body use glucose and secrete insulin.
- Brown rice provides about fourteen percent of your daily need for fiber, which helps reduce high cholesterol, fight atherosclerosis, prevent constipation and diverticulosis, and avoid colon cancer. Fiber also helps keep blood sugar levels under control.
- The oil in whole brown rice lowers cholesterol levels.
- A study published in the *American Journal of Gastroenterology* shows that eating foods high in insoluble fiber, such as brown rice, can help women avoid gallstones.

How to Select and Store

Choose organic brown rice when possible. Unlike white rice, brown rice has an oil-rich germ, which is susceptible to becoming rancid. Therefore, store brown rice in the refrigerator in an airtight container. It should stay fresh for about six months.

NUTTY BROWN RICE
Serves 4
2 Tbs olive oil
¼ cup chopped green onions
½ cup dried cranberries
1 cup brown rice, uncooked
2½ cups vegetable broth
1 cup chopped pecans

Heat oil in a deep skillet or saucepan and add onions. Sauté until soft. Add the cranberries, rice, and broth. Cook covered for 45 minutes. To serve, add the pecans and stir.

MEXICAN BROWN RICE
Serves 8
2 Tbs olive oil
2 cups brown rice, uncooked
3 cups vegetable broth
1½ cups finely chopped onion
2 tsp minced garlic
1 can (14 oz) Mexican-style tomatoes
1 bell pepper, chopped fine
Salt and pepper to taste

Heat oil in a nonstick saucepan over medium heat and sauté the rice until golden (about 5 minutes). Add ½ cup of broth if needed, then add the onions and garlic and sauté for a few minutes. Stir in tomatoes (with juice), remaining broth, and bell pepper. Bring to a boil, reduce heat and simmer, covered, for 20–25 minutes or until broth is absorbed. Add salt and pepper if desired, and serve.

BUCKWHEAT

Most people think buckwheat is a grain, and it does have some wheatlike characteristics, but it is actually a fruit seed related to rhubarb. That's good news for people who are allergic or sensitive to wheat and other glutinous grains, because buckwheat is gluten-free. That means you can eat all the buckwheat pancakes you want!

Buckwheat is native to Northern Europe and Asia, and was introduced to the United States by the Dutch during the seventeenth century. Today it is produced primarily in Poland and Russia, as well as the United States, Canada, and France. Buckwheat is sold either roasted (called "kasha" or "groats") or unroasted. Unroasted buckwheat has a subtle flavor, while roasted buckwheat has a nutty taste. It is often ground into flour and can be used for baking and for making pancakes and crepes.

Buckwheat Nutrition
Serving Size: ½ cup roasted, dry (kasha)
Calories: 284
Protein: 9.6 g
Total Fat: 2.2 g
Carbohydrates: 61.5 g
Fiber: 8.4 g
Cholesterol: 0 mg
Copper: 0.5 mg, 55% DRI
Iron: 2 mg, 15% DRI
Magnesium: 181 mg, 47% DRI
Manganese: 1.3 mg, 65% DRI
Zinc: 2 mg, 22% DRI

Health Benefits
Buckwheat has a lot going for it: besides being a great alternative for wheat, it is also rich in fiber, magnesium, and special flavonoids that protect against disease. It is also a source of high-quality protein, as it contains all eight essential amino acids. Let's look at this "grain."

- A study of more than 800 people who consumed a diet high in buckwheat (about 3.5 oz. daily) had improved total cholesterol, low-density lipoprotein (LDL) cholesterol, and high-density lipoprotein (HDL) cholesterol levels.
- The flavonoids in buckwheat, especially rutin and quercitin, boost the antioxidant benefits of vitamin C, help maintain blood flow, prevent platelets from excessive clotting, and hinder oxidation of LDL cholesterol, all of which protect against cardiovascular conditions, including atherosclerosis, heart attack, and stroke.
- The magnesium in buckwheat can lower blood pressure by relaxing blood vessels and thus enhancing

blood flow and delivery of nutrients throughout the body.

- A Canadian study found that buckwheat seed extract lowered blood glucose levels by up to nineteen percent in lab animals. The substance in buckwheat responsible for this benefit is chiro-inositol, which has played a role in glucose metabolism in human studies.

- A study in *American Journal of Gastroenterology* reports that foods high in insoluble fiber, such as buckwheat, can help prevent gallstones in women. Experts believe insoluble fiber speeds up transit time, reduces the secretion of bile acids, and lowers triglyceride levels.

- A large (six hundred participants) Dutch study found that children who ate a significant amount of whole grains were fifty-four percent less likely to be asthmatic than those who ate a low amount.

- Numerous studies show that diets high in fiber-rich whole grains, including buckwheat, carry a lower risk of colon cancer.

How to Select and Store

Buckwheat is available in bulk bins and in packages. In either form, make sure the buckwheat has not been exposed to moisture. At home, store buckwheat in an airtight container and keep it in a cool, dry place. Buckwheat flour should always be refrigerated. Buckwheat groats are best refrigerated if you live in a warm climate. If stored properly, buckwheat will keep for up to one year; buckwheat flour will stay fresh for several months.

KASHI CHILI

Serves 4

1 28-oz can stewed tomatoes
3 cups vegetable broth
1 15-oz can pinto or black beans
1 tsp each: cumin, ground oregano, minced garlic
1 Tbs chili powder
¾ cup buckwheat (uncooked)

In a large skillet, bring the tomatoes, broth, and spices to a boil for 10 minutes. Add the buckwheat and beans, cover and simmer for 10–15 minutes, or until kasha is tender. Serve.

BUCKWHEAT PANCAKES
Serves 4
1 cup buckwheat flour
1 tsp baking powder
2 Tbs sugar
1 egg, beaten
1 cup nonfat milk
2 Tbs melted margarine or canola oil

Preheat a lightly greased skillet. Mix the dry ingredients together, then add the egg, milk, and margarine, mixing well. Pour ¼ cup of batter onto the hot skillet. Cook until the bubbles break on the surface, then turn and bake an additional 1 to 1½ minutes.

BULGAR

Bulgar, bulghur, burghul . . . no matter how you spell it, bulgar wheat is delicious and nutritious. This Middle Eastern staple food is often confused with cracked wheat, and while the two are similar in consistency and texture, bulgar is lower in fat and has more nutrients than cracked wheat. Bulgar is wheat kernels that have been steamed, dried, and crushed. Its nutty flavor can be enjoyed alone or in many recipes.

Bulgar Nutrition
Serving Size: 1 cup cooked
Calories: 151
Protein: 6 g
Total Fat: 0 g
Carbohydrates: 34 g
Fiber: 8 g
Cholesterol: 0 mg

Copper: 0.13 mg, 14% DRI
Iron: 1.7 mg, 13% DRI
Magnesium: 58 mg, 15% DRI
Manganese: 1.1 mg, 55% DRI
Niacin: 1.8 mg, 12% DRI
Thiamin: 0.1 mg, 8% DRI
Vitamin B-6: 0.15 mg, 10% DRI
Zinc: 1 mg, 11% DRI

Health Benefits

We're not saying other grains aren't nutritious; they are. But bulgar has less fat and higher levels of most nutrients than many of its cousins. The benefits to your health can be considerable!

- Bulgar contains phytonutrients known as lignans, which help keep the blood vessels healthy and protect against atherosclerosis, heart attack, and stroke.
- The high fiber content in bulgar goes a long way toward preventing and/or treating various cancers (especially colon cancer), constipation, diabetes (type 2), diventricular disease, heart disease, hemorrhoids, high cholesterol, hypertension, irritable bowel syndrome, obesity, stroke, and varicose veins.
- A Harvard study shows that women who consumed the most whole grains like bulgar were about twenty-five percent less likely to develop type 2 diabetes than those who ate a less varied diet.
- Eating an average of 2.5 servings of whole grains, like bulgar, daily is associated with a 21 percent lower risk of heart disease.
- Bulgar is a good source of nutrients that help with symptoms of PMS and menopause, including magnesium, manganese, vitamin B-6, and complex carbohydrates.
- Bulgar contains lutein (72 mg per 1 cup cooked), a phytonutrient that helps prevent cataracts, macular degeneration, and glaucoma.

• People with rheumatoid arthritis, diabetes, or osteoporosis may benefit from consuming manganese, which is present in high levels in bulgar.

How to Select and Store

Bulgar is usually found in bulk-food sections or in supermarkets near the rice or specialty foods, and is often labeled "tabbouleh." Choose organic bulgar when possible. Store the grain in an airtight container and keep in a cool, dry place. Bulgar keeps for up to six months in the refrigerator or at room temperature, and for many months longer in the freezer.

BULGAR SALAD

Serves 6
¾ cup dry bulgar
1⅓ cup water
1 tsp salt
1 cup corn, fresh cut from cob or frozen (thawed)
1 Tbs olive oil
1 pint cherry tomatoes, halved
2 Tbs red wine vinegar
1 tsp pepper
⅓ cup chopped scallions

In a large skillet, toast bulgar over medium heat for 5–10 minutes, stirring occasionally until browned. Add water and salt and bring to a boil. Reduce heat and simmer covered for 5–10 minutes or until water is absorbed. Remove from heat and let stand 10 minutes covered. Transfer to bowl and cool in refrigerator. In the meantime, sauté the corn in oil for 5–7 minutes. Cool. Add corn, tomatoes, scallions, vinegar and pepper to bulgar. Toss and chill before serving.

BULGAR RAISIN PILAF

Serves 4
1⅓ cup bulgar
1⅓ cup boiling water
4 Tbs raisins

¼ tsp salt
¼ tsp ground cumin

Place bulgar in a medium-size bowl and cover with boiling
water. Add remaining ingredients and stir well. Let stand 30
minutes until water is absorbed.

CABBAGE

Cabbage is a member of the cruciferous family, which is also
populated by broccoli, cauliflower, radishes, and other vegetables whose leaves grow at right angles to each other, forming
a cross (crucifer). Cabbage is also one of the oldest cultivated
vegetables. It was enjoyed by the ancient Romans both as a
food and as a medicine to treat wounds, colic, and to prevent
plague. In later centuries other cultures used it to treat bruises,
poisoning, dog bites, and acne. Today, experts have analyzed
cabbage and identified the substances that make it such an important vegetable to include in your diet. With more than 400
varieties to choose from, you could try a new one each day for
more than a year!

Cabbage Nutrition
Serving Size for All: 1 cup, chopped and cooked

Green Cabbage
Calories: 39
Protein: 2 g
Total Fat: 0 g
Carbohydrates: 8 g
Fiber: 2.8 g
Cholesterol: 0 mg
Vitamin C: 56 mg, 68% DRI
Potassium: 294 mg, 6% DRI
Folate: 44 mcg, 11% DRI

Red Cabbage
Calories: 44
Protein: 2 g
Total Fat: 0 g
Carbohydrates: 10 g
Fiber: 3.8 g
Cholesterol: 0 mg
Vitamin C: 51 mg, 62% DRI
Vitamin B-6: 0.338 mg, 23% DRI
Folate: 36 mcg, 9% DRI
Potassium: 392 mg, 8% DRI
Iron: 1 mg, 8% DRI

Bok Choy
Calories: 20
Protein: 1.3 g
Total Fat: 0 g
Carbohydrates: 3 g
Fiber: 1.7 g
Cholesterol: 0 mg
Vitamin A: 3612 IU, 138% DRI
Vitamin C: 44 mg, 53% DRI
Potassium: 631 mg, 14% DRI
Iron: 1.7 mg, 13% DRI
Calcium: 158 mg, 16% DRI

Health Benefits
Although each variety of cabbage differs somewhat in nutritional value, they all provide healthy levels of vitamin C and various phytonutrients, including flavonoids, indoles, and sulforaphane. Here's a closer look.

- The indoles in cabbage may help prevent breast cancer by converting estradiol, an estrogen-like hormone, into a safer form of estrogen.
- The sulforaphane and indole-3-carbinol in cabbage have been shown to help the liver rid itself of toxins, and to prevent cancer.

- Vitamin C is a potent antioxidant that supports the immune system and helps fight bacterial and viral infections, including the common cold, bronchitis, and ear infections.
- If you don't eat dairy products (and even if you do), bok choy is a good source of calcium, which helps prevent osteoporosis and control high blood pressure.
- Cabbage contains sulfur and histidine, substances that can strengthen the immune system and reduce tumor growth.
- Cabbage can heal ulcers, as it contains the amino acid L-glutamine, which protects the stomach lining, and gefarnate, a substance that stimulates the secretion of mucus from the stomach's lining. Studies show that drinking thirty-two ounces of cabbage juice daily (from green cabbage) can help heal ulcers.
- When cabbage is chewed, anticancer substances called glucosinolates and myrosinase are released.

How to Select and Store

Look for heads that are solid and heavy for their size, and leaves that are not wilted. Store cabbage in a plastic bag in the refrigerator crisper section, where it should keep for one week or longer.

RED, WHITE, AND GREEN SALAD
Serves 2
¼ medium green cabbage, cut into pieces
½ small red bell pepper, cut into pieces
1 small white onion, chopped
½ tsp olive oil
1 Tbs low-salt soy sauce

Combine vegetables in a bowl. Whisk together the oil and soy sauce and mix into vegetables.

CABBAGE SOUP
Serves 3–4
1 tsp olive oil

1 onion, minced
3½ cups vegetable broth
2 oz whole wheat noodles
½ head green or red cabbage, shredded
1 tsp dry sherry

In a skillet, heat the oil, add onion and cook about 1 minute over low heat. Add the broth and noodles, raise heat and bring to a boil. Boil for 5 minutes. Reduce heat and add cabbage and simmer 5 minutes. Stir in sherry and serve.

CARROT

Caucus carota, or the carrot, is a crunchy, mildly sweet vegetable that belongs to the same family as cumin, dill, fennel, and parsnips. Carrots were originally lavender to deep purple, and were cultivated in the Middle East and central Asia thousands of years ago. A yellow variety likely got its start in Afghanistan and was later adopted by the ancient Romans and Greeks. Around the seventeenth century the orange carrot seen today was first cultivated in Europe by agriculturists who wanted a carrot that had a better texture than the purple variety. Although purple, white, yellow, and black carrots are still grown today, orange varieties are the most popular.

Carrot Nutrition
Serving Size: 1 large (7¼–8½")
Calories: 30
Protein: 0.5 g
Total Fat: 0 g
Carbohydrates: 7 g
Fiber: 2 g
Cholesterol: 0 mg
Vitamin A: 12,028 IU, 460% DRI

Health Benefits

Carrots are an excellent source of antioxidants, including ly-copene, lutein, and zeaxanthin, and especially the carotenoids, featuring beta-carotene as the star nutrient: one cup of carrots provides more than 16,000 IUs, or about 685 percent of the DRI, for vitamin A. Let's look at this colorful vegetable.

- Eating at least one serving of carrots per day may re-duce your risk of heart attack by sixty percent, accord-ing to one study.
- Beta-carotene, lutein, and zeaxanthin protect the eyes against cataracts and macular degeneration. The liver converts the beta-carotene in carrots to vitamin A and sends it to the retina.
- A high intake of carotenoids is associated with a twenty percent decrease in postmenopausal breast can-cer and a decrease in cancer of the bladder, cervix, colon, esophagus, larynx, and prostate.
- Carrots may fight asthma in children. Results of a large 2004 study found that children who had higher blood levels of beta-carotene, vitamin C, and selenium were ten to twenty percent less likely to develop asthma than their peers.
- The antioxidants in carrots fight inflammation, which can reduce the symptoms of arthritis, fibromyalgia, and other inflammatory conditions.
- Antioxidants are a great boost to the immune system in helping fight bacterial and viral infections, includ-ing bronchitis, the common cold, ear infections, and urinary tract infections.

How to Select and Store

Look for carrots that are firm, smooth, and bright in color. If the tops are attached, look for feathery, bright greens. If the tops have been removed, the stem end should not be dark, as this is a sign of age. To preserve freshness, store carrots in the coolest part of the refrigerator in a plastic bag or wrapped in paper towels. Cut off the green tops before storing, and keep carrots away from fruits because most of them produce ethylene gas (vegetables to a lesser extent) that will make the carrots bitter. Carrots typically will stay relatively fresh for two weeks if stored properly.

ZESTY CARROT SOUP
Serves 4–6
8 carrots, chopped
4 celery stalks, chopped
2 cloves garlic, chopped
1 medium red onion, chopped
1 small red pepper, chopped fine
4 cups water
1 Tbs olive oil
1 tsp curry powder

Heat the olive oil in a skillet, add the garlic and onion and sauté for 4–5 minutes. Add the curry powder and stir. Add all remaining ingredients and cook until the vegetables are tender. Place the vegetable mixture into a blender and process until it reaches desired consistency. Add salt if desired and serve.

GARLIC CARROTS
Serves 6
1 lb baby carrots
2 cloves garlic, minced
2 Tbs olive oil
½ cup celery, chopped
¼ cup hot water
½ tsp salt
¼ tsp dried thyme

In a skillet, sauté the carrots, celery, and garlic in oil for 5 minutes. Add water, salt, thyme, and pepper. Bring to a boil, reduce heat, cover, and cook for 8–12 minutes or until carrots are tender.

CANTALOUPE

Did you know that the melon with the distinctly webbed rind that Americans call a cantaloupe is not a true cantaloupe, but a muskmelon? Real cantaloupes are grown in Europe and have deep grooves in the rind. However, we talk here about the muskmelon-known-as-a-cantaloupe and reveal some of its healthful qualities.

Cantaloupes were believed to be cultivated first in Egypt and then carried to Iran, India, and beyond during biblical times. Their popularity spread quickly and continued through the millennia. The "cantaloupe" we are familiar with today was first sent to the United States by the French in 1881. It was developed by W. Atlee Burpee Company and given the name Netted Gem because of the netted appearance of the rind. Although it was first grown commercially in Colorado, today around seventy percent of cantaloupes in the United States are grown in California.

Cantaloupe Nutrition
Serving Size: 1 cup diced
Calories: 53
Protein: 1 g
Total Fat: 0 g
Carbohydrates: 12.7 g
Fiber: 1.4 g
Cholesterol: 0 mg
Vitamin A: 5276 IU, 202% DRI
Vitamin C: 57 mg, 70% DRI
Folate: 33 mcg, 8% DRI
Potassium: 417 mg, 9% DRI

Health Benefits
Cantaloupe provides high levels of vitamin C and beta-carotene/vitamin A, and it's low in calories. If you are trying to lose weight, cantaloupe is a great sweet treat that doesn't add on pounds. But cantaloupe has many other healthful benefits as well.

- The potassium in cantaloupe can help lower blood pressure.
- Cantaloupe is heart-friendly: the vitamin C protects against the formation of blood clots, which helps prevent atherosclerosis, heart attack, stroke, and other cardiovascular conditions.
- Vision problems, including cataracts and macular degeneration, are targeted by beta-carotene and vitamin C.
- The powerful combination of vitamin A/beta-carotene and vitamin C in cantaloupe may help prevent and/or treat acne, bursitis, constipation, eczema, gingivitis, herpes, shingles, ulcers, and urinary tract infections.

How to Select and Store

May through October is harvest time for California cantaloupe, with imports from South America much of the remaining year. When choosing a cantaloupe, look for a rind that is slightly golden. The stem end should have a slight indentation. The blossom end should be slightly soft when gently pressed and should smell sweet when the melon is at room temperature.

To ripen a cantaloupe, leave it at room temperature for 2 to 4 days. Watch it carefully, as cantaloupe can ripen very quickly. Once it reaches desired softness, refrigerate it, where it should remain good for up to 14 days uncut, less time once it is cut.

CANTALOUPE SMOOTHIE
Makes 4 cups
½ ripe cantaloupe, peeled and cut into chunks
1 cup vanilla soymilk
1 cup vanilla fat-free yogurt
1 cup crushed ice

Place all ingredients into a blender and process until smooth.

STUFFED PASTA SHELLS
Serves 3
6 oz cooked turkey breast

6 jumbo pasta shells
1 medium mango, peeled and chopped
½ medium cantaloupe, seeded and diced
¼ cup nonfat sour cream
1 Tbs fresh chives, minced
2 Tbs lime juice
1 tsp Dijon mustard
Salt and pepper

Cut cooked turkey breast into pieces. Cook pasta according to package directions. Rinse the cooked shells in cold water and set aside. Combine the mango, cantaloupe, turkey, and remaining ingredients. Stuff the shells with the mixture. Serve at room temperature or chilled.

CAULIFLOWER

"Cabbage flower"—that's the translation of the Latin terms *caulis* (cabbage) and *floris* (flower) from which "cauliflower" was born. The oldest record of cauliflower comes from the sixth century BC, and it was noted by European writers in the sixteenth century. Today this popular cruciferous vegetable is grown mainly in Salinas Valley in California.

Cauliflower Nutrition
Serving Size: 1 cup, 1 inch pieces
Calories: 28
Protein: 2 g
Total Fat: 0.5 g
Carbohydrates 5 g
Fiber: 2.5 g
Cholesterol: 0 mg
Vitamin C: 55 mg, 67% DRI
Folate: 54 mcg, 13% DRI
Vitamin B-6: 0.214 mg, 14% DRI

Health Benefits

As one of the cruciferous vegetables, cauliflower is associated with cancer-fighting properties, but the benefits don't stop there. Let's talk cauliflower.

- Cauliflower contains allicin, a substance also found in onions and garlic, which helps prevent heart attack, stroke, and other cardiovascular ailments.
- Cauliflower is a good source of both vitamin C and selenium, two antioxidants that support the immune system and help fight infections such as the common cold, flu, sinusitis, and bronchitis.
- The phytonutrients sulforaphane and isothiocyanate, among others, in cauliflower enhance the ability of the liver to neutralize toxic substances that can cause cancer. Cauliflower also contains detoxifying enzymes, including glutathione transferase and quinine reductase. Studies show that cruciferous vegetables like cauliflower reduce the risk of lung, colon, breast, bladder, and ovarian cancer.
- Cauliflower contains indole-3-carbinol, a phytonutrient that impacts estrogen and can help prevent breast and other hormone-related cancers.
- Cauliflower provides fiber, which can help reduce the risk of colon cancer and prevent constipation, diverticulitis, and other intestinal ailments.
- A large study shows that children with asthma who consume a diet high in vitamin C experience less wheezing than children who don't follow such a diet.

How to Select and Store

Choose cauliflower that is firm, heavy for its size, and whose curd (flower head) is tight and unblemished. Refrigerate the head stem-side up and store it in an open or perforated plastic bag. Cauliflower will keep for up to five days if stored in the crisper drawer in the refrigerator, but for best flavor eat as soon as possible. Precut florets should be eaten the same day they are purchased.

BAKED CAULIFLOWER
Serves 4
1 head cauliflower
2 cloves garlic, minced
2 Tbs olive oil
1 lemon
Salt and pepper
Grated cheese if desired

Preheat oven to 400° F. Lightly oil a shallow ovenproof casserole dish. Cut cauliflower into florets and put in a single layer in the casserole. Sprinkle with minced garlic. Squeeze the juice of a lemon over the cauliflower. Drizzle each piece with olive oil and sprinkle with salt and pepper. Place in the oven, uncovered, for 10–15 minutes or until the top is lightly browned. Sprinkle with grated cheese.

RED, WHITE, & GREEN SAUTÉ
Serves 4
2 cups fresh cauliflower florets
½ cup sliced onion
½ cup diced celery
1 clove garlic, minced
1 Tbs olive oil
1 cup fresh or frozen snow pea pods
1 red bell pepper, cut into strips
½ cup sliced fresh mushrooms
1 tsp dried oregano
¼ tsp salt

Steam cauliflower in a steamer basket, drain, and set aside. Cook onion, garlic, and celery in olive oil in a large skillet over medium heat, stirring constantly until tender. Add cauliflower, snow peas, and remaining ingredients, stirring constantly until heated.

CELERY

What we know as celery today is believed to be the same plant Homer mentioned in his *Odyssey* about 850 BC. Homer's *selinon* most likely became *celery* by way of the French *celery*, which is derived from ancient Greek. Celery was originally used only for medicinal purposes, mainly as a diuretic and to reduce blood pressure. It wasn't until 1623 in France that its use as food was first recorded. It did not become popular until the eighteenth century in Europe, and not until the early nineteenth century in America.

Celery Nutrition
Serving Size: 1 cup, cooked, no salt
Calories: 27
Protein: 1.25 g
Total Fat: 0 g
Carbohydrates: 6 g
Fiber: 2.4 g
Cholesterol: 0 mg
Potassium: 426 mg, 9% AI
Magnesium: 18 mg, 5% DRI
Calcium: 63 mg, 6% DRI
Vitamin C: 9.2 mg, 11% DRI

Health Benefits
Celery's main nutritional claims revolve around its vitamin C content and several potent phytonutrients. Let's look at them.

- Celery contains phthalides, which can help reduce high blood pressure. They do this by relaxing the muscles around arteries, which dilates the arteries and allows blood to flow more efficiently. Phthalides also reduce the level of stress hormones, which cause blood vessels to relax.
- Another compound in celery is coumarins, which may work to prevent cancer.

- Celery is a good source of potassium, calcium, and magnesium, all of which help reduce blood pressure by stimulating urine production and eliminating excess fluid from the body.
- Celery may lower cholesterol by increasing the secretion of bile, a substance that removes cholesterol from the body.

How to Select and Store

Select celery that looks crisp, tight, and snaps easily when you pull the stalks apart. The leaves should be pale to bright green, not yellow or brown. Gently inspect between the stalks to see if there is insect damage known as "blackheart," which appears as brown or black discoloration. Store celery in a sealed container or wrap it in a damp cloth or plastic bag and refrigerate it. Cut or peeled celery should be stored free from any moisture. Do not freeze celery unless you plan to use it in a cooked recipe.

GREEN, BLACK, AND RED SALAD
Serves 2
1 bunch celery
4 radishes, trimmed and cut into slices
10 pitted black olives, chopped
1 Tbs virgin olive oil
1 Tbs chopped fresh chives
2 tsp lemon juice
⅛ tsp each salt and black pepper

Remove outer dark ribs of the celery and reserve for soup. Remove leaves and place in a bowl. Cut remaining stalks into ¼-inch slices and add to leaves. Add remaining ingredients and toss. Chill before serving.

CELERY BEAN SOUP
Serves 4
2 Tbs olive oil
1 onion, chopped

4 celery stalks, chopped
3 cloves garlic, minced
32 oz white or pink beans, cooked and drained
2 cups vegetable bouillon

Sauté the onion and celery in the oil until transparent. Add the beans and bouillon and cook on low heat for 15 minutes. Puree to desired consistency. Garnish with croutons.

CINNAMON

For many people, a whiff of cinnamon evokes thoughts of apple pie and cider—warm, comfortable feelings. Cinnamon has been stirring up good feelings for millennia: it was used in ancient Egypt as medicine and as a beverage flavoring, and, in a less-pleasant way, as an embalming ingredient, while the Chinese mentioned it in their botanical medicine books as long ago as 2700 BC. Cinnamon's popularity continues today, both as a food and beverage favorite and, increasingly, to treat medical conditions. It is grown mainly in Sri Lanka, India, Brazil, and the Caribbean.

Cinnamon Nutrition
Serving Size: 1 Tbs
Calories: 19
Protein: 0.3 g
Total Fat: 0 g
Carbohydrates: 6 g
Fiber: 4 g
Cholesterol: 0 mg
Calcium: 78 mg, 7.8% DRI
Manganese: 1.36 mg, 68% AI

Health Benefits
Cinnamon has healing abilities that can be attributed to several basic components found in the essential oils: cinnamaldehyde, cinnamyl acetate, and cinnamyl alcohol.

- Cinnamaldehyde helps prevent unwanted clotting of blood by inhibiting the release of arachidonic acid. This action also reduces inflammation.
- Cinnamon slows the rate at which the stomach empties after eating, which reduces the rise in blood glucose levels and thus is helpful for type 2 diabetes.
- Cinnamon can improve cognitive skills, including memory and attention, according to preliminary research presented by Dr. Zoladz at the 2004 meeting of the Association for Chemoreception Sciences. This benefit comes from chewing cinnamon gum or simply smelling the spice.
- Several studies show that some of cinnamon's components fight bacterial and yeast infections, including *Candida*, *Enterobacter*, *Staphylococcus*, and *Escherichia coli*.
- This remedy for diarrhea is anecdotal but many people swear by it: steep 1 tablespoon of cinnamon in 8 ounces of hot water for 10 minutes. Have several cups per day.

How to Select and Store

Cinnamon is available in powder or stick form. Ground cinnamon has a more potent flavor than the stick. Ground cinnamon should be stored in a tightly sealed glass container in a dark, cool place, where it will keep for about six months. Cinnamon sticks usually stay fresh for about one year if stored in a similar way. Refrigerating cinnamon will extend the life even longer. To check the freshness of cinnamon, smell it: if it smells sweet, it's fresh; if not, it's stale.

CINNAMON TIPS

- Sprinkle one teaspoon on oatmeal.
- Blend one or two teaspoons into a vanilla smoothie.
- Sprinkle cinnamon on apple and pear slices.
- Add cinnamon to mashed sweet potatoes, yams, pumpkin, or squash dishes.

CINNAMON BANANAS

Serves 4

3 bananas, quartered
½ tsp orange zest
1 tsp lime juice
½ cup orange juice
¼ cup raisins
¼ tsp vanilla extract
¼ tsp cinnamon

Preheat oven to 375F. Place bananas in a single layer in a baking dish. Combine all remaining ingredients and pour over bananas. Bake 15–20 minutes.

CRANBERRIES

Cranberries are one of the three native North American fruits (blueberries and Concord grapes are the other two). Native Americans used the cranberry for medicinal purposes as well as for food, and as a dye. Early American mariners brought cranberries with them on their ships to prevent scurvy, as they are a great source of vitamin C. Around 1610–1616, Captain Henry Hall was the first American to successfully cultivate cranberries, and thanks to him we are enjoying US-grown cranberries today.

Cranberry Nutrition

Serving Size: 1 cup, whole, raw
Calories: 46
Protein: 0.4 g
Total Fat: 0.2 g
Carbohydrates: 12 g
Fiber: 4.6 g
Cholesterol: 0 mg
Vitamin C: 13 mg, 16% DRI

Health Benefits

Cranberries contain some very important nutrients, including proanthocyanidins, which prevent the activities of certain bacteria, and antioxidants, which fight free radicals that can cause serious diseases.

- The proanthocyanidins in cranberries have been shown to effectively prevent and treat urinary tract infections by preventing *E. coli*, the bacteria associated with such infections, from sticking to the urinary tract walls.
- Proanthocyanidins found in cranberry juice prevent the adhesion of *Helicobacter pylori*, the bacteria associated with stomach ulcers, to the stomach wall.
- Cranberries fight the buildup of plaque, which causes gingivitis.
- Cranberries contain flavonoids and other phytonutrients that can protect against atherosclerosis by inhibiting the damage caused by low-density lipoprotein (LDL) cholesterol.

How to Select and Store

Look for cranberries that are bright and plump. When you get them home, refrigerate them immediately, unwashed, as moisture will cause them to spoil quickly. Properly stored cranberries should keep up to eight weeks in the refrigerator. They can also be stored in the freezer: place them unwashed in a plastic bag for freezing.

SAUTÉ CRANBERRIES AND CARROTS

Serves 4–6

1 lb carrots, cut into 3" × ½" sticks
1 tsp salt
1 tsp cinnamon
¾ tsp dry mustard
¼ cup orange juice
2 Tbs butter
½ cup dried cranberries
⅓ cup pecans, chopped

In a large saucepan, place carrots and ½ tsp salt, cover with water, and bring to a boil. Reduce heat and cook until the carrots are tender, about 10 minutes. Drain and place in a bowl. In another bowl, combine the cinnamon, mustard and remaining salt and stir in orange juice. Melt butter in the saucepan, add the carrots and orange juice mixture. Cook 2–3 minutes, then add the cranberries and heat through. Garnish with pecans.

CRANBERRY TWIST
Serves 1
6 oz unsweetened cranberry juice
2 oz orange juice
2 oz seltzer water

Combine all ingredients and enjoy.

DARK CHOCOLATE

Is this too good to be true? Is dark chocolate a healthful food? Yes, in moderation. Dark chocolate contains much more cocoa than other types of chocolate, and the cocoa is the ingredient that harbors the beneficial nutrients.

Cocoa, or cacao, comes from the *Theobroma cacao* tree, which literally means "food of the gods." Cacao originated in Latin America, but Africa is the major producer of cocoa today. The world's leading consumer of cocoa is the United States.

Dark Chocolate Nutrition
Serving Size: 1 ounce semisweet
Calories: 134
Protein: 1.2 g
Total Fat: 7.3 g
Carbohydrates: 18.5 g
Fiber: 2 g
Cholesterol: 0 mg
Iron: 0.81 mg, 6% DRI

Serving Size: 1 ounce unsweetened, baking
Calories: 140
Protein: 3.6 g
Total Fat: 14.6 g
Carbohydrates: 8.3 g
Fiber: 4.6 g
Cholesterol: 0 mg
Iron: 4.87 mg, 37% DRI
Copper: 0.9 mg, 100% DRI
Zinc: 2.7 mg, 30% DRI
Magnesium: 92 mg, 24% DRI

Health Benefits

The health benefits from dark chocolate come from the cocoa, which contains phenols, a class of phytonutrients. Although milk chocolate also contains cocoa, the milk and sugar cancel out the benefits of the cocoa, while the manufacturing process removes most of the flavonoids. Unsweetened baking chocolate offers more nutrients than processed dark chocolate.

• The phenols in dark chocolate are a powerful antioxidant and can reduce high blood pressure. Eating two to three ounces of dark chocolate daily can lead to this result. To offset the high calories and fat, you should reduce and/or eliminate other high-fat, high-calorie items from your diet.
• The flavonoids in dark chocolate can help prevent atherosclerosis and heart disease, as they prevent blood platelets from sticking together and causing clots.

How to Select and Store

Look for organic dark chocolate with a minimum of 70% chocolate solids. The most nutritious dark chocolates are unsweetened and semisweet. Chocolate should be stored in a dry, cool place. If you need to refrigerate it because of high temperatures, place it in an airtight container to prevent exposure to moisture and odors, as chocolate is very susceptible to picking up odors from other foods.

CHOCOLATE-COVERED STRAWBERRIES
15 large strawberries with stems attached
3 oz bittersweet dark chocolate
2 Tbs half and half
2 tsp brandy

Line a baking or cookie sheet with waxed paper. Wash strawberries and dry thoroughly. Strawberries should be at room temperature when dipping. Prepare chocolate in one of two ways: (1) in a double boiler over hot water, melt chocolate. Add half and half and stir until smooth. Remove from heat and blend in brandy. Let the chocolate cool slightly before dipping. (2) In a microwave-safe bowl, melt chocolate. Remove from microwave and stir until smooth. Blend in half and half and brandy. For each strawberry, grasp the stem and dip the fruit into the chocolate, swirl, and shake as you withdraw the strawberry. Place on the prepared baking sheet. Refrigerate for about 30 minutes.

CHOCOLATE APPETIZERS
1 baguette loaf, cut into ¼-inch slices
Semisweet chocolate squares
Extra virgin olive oil
Coarse sea salt

Preheat the oven to 350 degrees F. Place the baguette slices on an ungreased baking sheet. Top each slice with a thin square of semisweet chocolate. The chocolate should be smaller than the slice. Bake the slices until the chocolate is melted but still keeps its shape. Remove from the oven and place on a serving dish. Sprinkle each slice with a few drops of olive oil, then add a tiny dash of salt to each slice.

EGGS

Archaeologists have found evidence that our ancestors from the Neolithic age enjoyed eggs as part of their diet. They also discovered that jungle fowl were domesticated by people in India by 3200 BC, and that the Egyptians and Chinese had domesticated fowl for eggs around 1400 BC. Domesticated fowl made the trip to North America with Columbus on his second journey in 1493, and people in the United States have been enjoying eggs ever since then.

Egg Nutrition

Serving Size: 1 large egg, hard boiled
Calories: 78
Protein: 6.3 g
Total Fat: 5.3 g
Carbohydrates: 0.5 g
Fiber: 0 g
Cholesterol: 212 mg
Selenium: 15.4 mcg, 28% DRI
Vitamin B-12: 0.56, 23% DRI
Riboflavin: 0.257 mcg, 11% DRI
Vitamin D: 18 IU, 4.5% DRI

Health Benefits

Many people consider eggs to be taboo because of their cholesterol content, but recent research indicates that eating eggs raises HDL (the good cholesterol) levels. What other benefits do eggs offer?

- Results of a 2006 study show that when people ate three or more eggs daily, they produced larger LDL (low-density lipoprotein) and HDL particles than people who did not eat eggs. Earlier studies showed that larger LDL particles are less likely than small ones to cause cholesterol buildup in the arteries, and that larger HDL particles are more efficient at eliminating cholesterol from the body.
- Eggs can be instrumental in fighting obesity, because they are an excellent source of protein and very low in calories.

- The lutein and zeaxanthin in egg yolk are known to protect against macular degeneration and can be helpful in preventing cataracts, glaucoma, and other vision problems.
- Eggs are a good source of choline (about 112 mcg per egg yolk), which helps regulate brain health (and can help with memory), nervous system functioning, and cardiovascular health.

How to Select and Store

Eggs are classified according to a grading system, with AA being the most superior quality, followed by A and B. Since labeling isn't required, you may not see these designations, especially if you buy eggs from a farmers' market or private farmer.

You may want to choose eggs that have enhanced levels of omega-3 fatty acids. These come from hens fed a diet high in canola oil (as well as flaxseed and/or kelp) and contain about three times the amount of omega-3 fatty acids (100 mg) as a regular egg (37 mg). You must eat the yolks to get the omega-3s, however.

Choose eggs that are refrigerated and inspect them for cracks. Store eggs in the refrigerator in their original carton or another sealed container; do not store them on the refrigerator door. Eggs stored properly should stay fresh for about four weeks.

BAKED EGGS
Serves 4
6 eggs
3 Tbs chopped onion
¼ cup chopped green or red pepper
¼ cup bread crumbs
½ cup low-fat cheese, grated

Steam the onion and pepper in a small amount of water in a skillet and then place in a lightly greased baking dish. Break the eggs into the dish, keeping the yolks intact. Mix the crumbs and cheese together and sprinkle over the eggs. Bake in a 350° F oven until the eggs are set but not hard.

DEVILISH EGGS

Serves 6
6 hard-cooked eggs, cold
¼ cup plain low-fat yogurt
1 Tbs minced red pepper
1 tsp minced onion
1 tsp lemon juice
¼ tsp salt
¾ tsp prepared mustard

Cut the eggs in half lengthwise, remove the yolks and place them in a bowl. Mash yolks, add remaining ingredients and mix well. Refill the whites with the mixture and refrigerate or serve immediately.

FAT-FREE MILK

No one is sure exactly how long people have been drinking cow's milk, but experts estimate the practice began around 6,000 to 8,000 BC. The ancient Egyptians highly valued milk and other dairy foods, and around 500 AD people in Europe were especially fond of milk from both cows and sheep. Dairy cows were transported to America in the early seventeenth century, and unprocessed milk was the norm until the late nineteenth century, when pasteurization was introduced.

The Food and Drug Administration (FDA) has established standards for the different types of milk. Whole milk must have no less than 3.25 percent milk fat, while fat-free milk (also called skim milk) must have less than 0.5 percent milk fat.

Fat-Free Milk Nutrition

Serving Size: 8 ounces, with added vitamin A & protein fortified
Calories: 101

Protein: 9.7 g
Total Fat: 0.6 g
Carbohydrates: 13.68 g
Fiber: 0 g
Cholesterol: 5 mg
Calcium: 352 mg, 35% DRI
Vitamin A: 499 IU, 19% DRI
Vitamin D: 98 IU, 25% DRI
Riboflavin, 0.477 mg, 40% DRI
Vitamin B-12: 1.06 mcg, 44% DRI

Health Benefits

Fat-free milk, which contains only a very small amount of saturated fat as compared with low-fat and whole milk, can be a source of essential nutrients if you include dairy products in your diet. Here are some of those benefits:

- Low-fat milk is a very good source of calcium, vitamin D, vitamin K, and phosphorus—all necessary ingredients for bone health—and thus is a food that may help prevent osteoporosis.
- A very large study has shown that calcium can reduce symptoms of PMS.
- Several studies indicate that calcium may help obese adults lose weight, especially around the midsection
- Riboflavin and vitamin B-12 play important roles in energy production and in preventing fatigue, like that associated with chronic fatigue syndrome and fibromyalgia.
- Vitamin B-12 helps with red blood cell production, which can help prevent anemia.
- Vitamin A helps maintain the health of tissues that defend the body against invading infectious organisms that can cause bronchitis, the common cold, ear infections, and flu, among others.

How to Select and Store

Use the "sell-by" date to help you determine how long you will be able to safely use the milk. Milk that is properly refrigerated usually stays good for up to seven days after the "sell-by" date. Refrigerate the milk immediately when you get home, preferably in the back or coldest part of the refrigerator (not on the door). Always keep the milk container closed as milk easily absorbs aromas from other foods.

Nonfat milk is available in both fluid and dry forms and with added vitamins A and/or D and/or fortified with protein. Depending on which form you choose, the nutritional values will differ from those presented here.

CREAM OF BROCCOLI SOUP
Serves 4
3 cups fresh broccoli flowerets or 2 10-oz packages
   frozen broccoli
½ cup vegetable broth
1 Tbs margarine
1 Tbs all-purpose flour
½ tsp dried thyme
¼ tsp salt
1 cup nonfat milk

Steam the broccoli until tender. In a blender or food processor, combine broccoli and broth, blend until smooth. Melt margarine in a saucepan, stir in flour, thyme, and salt. Add milk and stir. Cook until slightly thickened. Stir in broccoli mixture and heat through, stirring constantly.

BERRY SMOOTHIE
Serves 1
1 cup nonfat milk
¾ cup berries (your choice)
½ tsp vanilla extract
3 ice cubes

Combine all ingredients in a blender or food processor, blend at high speed until frothy. Serve immediately.

FIGS

Figs are a nutritional bonanza: they have the highest mineral content of all common fruits. Figs are a member of the mulberry family and have been a favorite fruit since the earliest recorded history. It is believed they originated in Asia Minor and then spread throughout China, Egypt, Greece, and other Mediterranean countries. The Egyptians especially revered figs, and packed them into tombs to sustain the departed in the afterlife.

Figs were brought to England during the first half of the sixteenth century and to North America around 1790. Today the world's top producers of figs are Turkey, Egypt, and Greece. In the United States, ninety-eight percent of the figs are grown in California.

Fig Nutrition

Serving Size: 3 small raw figs
Calories: 90
Protein: 0.9 g
Total Fat: 0.36 g
Carbohydrates: 23 g
Fiber: 3.6 g
Cholesterol: 0 mg
Potassium: 279 mg, 6% DRI
Manganese, 0.153 mg, 7.6% DRI

Serving Size: 3 dried figs
Calories: 63
Protein: 0.84 g
Total Fat: 0.2 g
Carbohydrates: 16 g
Fiber: 2.5 g
Potassium: 171 mg, 3.6% DRI
Manganese: 0.129 mg, 6.4% DRI

Health Benefits

The high fiber, potassium, and manganese content of figs provide some delicious health benefits. Here are a few of them.

- If you are fortunate enough to find fig leaves, which are popular in some cultures, they have been shown to reduce the need for insulin in people who have type 1 diabetes.
- Including figs in your daily menu is a good way to avoid constipation, stay "regular," and help prevent intestinal disorders such as colitis, Crohn's disease, diverticular disease, and irritable bowel syndrome.
- Figs are a fair source of potassium, which helps reduce high blood pressure.
- Manganese is important in energy production, and thus can help fight symptoms of chronic fatigue syndrome and fibromyalgia; and it plays a role in bone growth, which makes it helpful in warding off osteoporosis.

How to Select and Store

More than 150 different varieties of figs are available, and they come in a wide range of colors and textures. Some of the more popular varieties include black mission (black/purple skin and pink flesh), kadota (green skin and purple flesh), calimyrna (green/yellow skin and amber flesh), and brown turkey (purple skin and red flesh). Most figs are sold dried, which means they can be enjoyed any time during the year. Fresh figs are highly perishable and will keep fresh only one to two days in the refrigerator. Because they bruise easily, they should be stored on a soft surface or wrapped to make sure they do not dry out. Dried figs will stay fresh for several months if they are well wrapped and kept in a cool, dark place or refrigerated. Select figs that are plump and tender and have a deep color with firm stems. They should smell mildly sweet and never sour.

STUFFED FIGS
10 large dried figs, soaked in brandy for 2 hours
2 oz slivered almonds
20 whole almonds
2 oz dark chocolate, chopped

Preheat oven to 350 F. Bake the slivered and whole almonds for 8–10 minutes until toasted. Remove from oven and cool. In a food processor, combine chocolate bits and slivered almonds, and process until coarsely chopped. With a small knife, open each fig and make a round cavity in each. Stuff each fig with the almond and chocolate mixture and place on a baking sheet with the opening on top. Bake 5 minutes. Do not overbake or the figs will become hard. Remove from oven and place two whole almonds in each opening, and serve warm.

FIG BUTTER
1 lb figs, stems removed
⅓ cup sugar
¼ cup port
1 Tbs lemon juice
2 tsp grated orange zest
Dash of vanilla extract

Place the figs in a blender and process to a pulp. Cook the pulp in a saucepan for about 30 minutes, stirring occasionally to prevent sticking. Add remaining ingredients and cook for an additional 15 minutes, stirring occasionally. Remove from heat and cool. Can be used as a spread or a dip for fruit.

FLAXSEED

The tiny seeds of the flax plant bear big benefits when it comes to health, and they taste good too! The flax plant has been around since the Stone Age, and there are records from ancient Greece of its use as a food. Charlemagne is responsible for encouraging the cultivation of flax in Europe, and the early colonists brought the plant to North America, including Canada, which is the world's leader in flax and flaxseed today.

Flaxseed Nutrition
Serving Size: 1 Tbs ground seeds
Calories: 37

Protein: 1.28 g
Total Fat: 2.95 g
Carbohydrates: 2 g
Fiber: 1.9 g
Cholesterol: 0 mg
Magnesium: 27 mg, 8% DRI

Serving Size: 1 Tbs whole seeds
Calories: 55
Protein: 1.88 g
Total Fat: 4.34 g
Carbohydrates: 2.97 g
Fiber: 2.8 g
Cholesterol: 0 mg
Magnesium: 40 mg, 15% DRI

Health Benefits

Flaxseeds are an excellent plant source of omega-3 fatty acids in the form of alpha-linolenic acid (ALA), which is converted into the omega-3 fatty acid called eicosapentaenoic acid (EPA). Flaxseed and flaxseed oil are good alternative sources of omega-3 fatty acids for anyone who does not eat fish and/or take fish oil supplements.

- Flaxseeds are a delicious way to help reduce the inflammation associated with arthritis, asthma, bursitis, fibromyalgia, migraine, osteoporosis, and PMS. One to three grams of flaxseed or one to three tablespoons of flaxseed oil daily are suggested.
- Flaxseed is a safe way to reduce cholesterol and triglyceride levels. One study found that patients with high cholesterol who ate twenty grams of flaxseed daily saw declines of seventeen percent in total cholesterol, thirty-six percent in triglycerides, and thirty-three percent in the ratio of total cholesterol. These results were similar to those seen in patients who took statin drugs, but the flaxseed users got their results drug-free and without side effects.

- Ground flaxseeds provide fiber that can reduce cholesterol levels in people who have atherosclerosis and heart disease. An *Archives of Internal Medicine* study reported that eating high-fiber foods such as flaxseed can help prevent heart disease.
- Fiber can help stabilize blood glucose levels in diabetics.
- The magnesium in flaxseeds can lower high blood pressure and help in the treatment of insomnia.
- Flaxseed contains lignans, substances which protect against development of breast cancer in women.
- One study found that among postmenopausal women who were suffering with hot flashes, 1.4 grams of flaxseed taken daily for six weeks reduced this symptom by nearly 60 percent.

How to Select and Store

Flaxseeds can be purchased as whole seeds or ground. Whole seeds should be stored in an airtight container and kept in a dark, dry, cool place, such as a refrigerator, and they will keep fresh for several months. If you buy ground flaxseeds, look for packages that are refrigerated or that are vacuum sealed, since ground seeds are prone to spoilage. Ground seeds can be stored in the refrigerator or freezer to prevent them from going rancid.

If you buy flaxseed oil, keep it refrigerated and in an opaque glass bottle. Flaxseed oil should not be used for cooking; instead drizzle it on prepared foods or on salads.

SUPER SMOOTHIE
Serves 1 or 2
1 cup orange juice
1 cup frozen berries (your choice)
1 ripe banana
2 Tbs ground flaxseed

Place all ingredients in a blender and process until smooth.

FLAX PANCAKES
Makes 6–8 pancakes
½ cup old-fashioned rolled oats
¾ cup whole wheat pancake mix
⅛ cup ground flaxseed
1 cup nonfat milk
1 egg

In a mixing bowl, combine all dry ingredients. Add milk and egg and stir until all dry ingredients are moistened. Let mixture stand for 15 minutes. Preheat lightly oiled griddle over medium heat. Pour a scant ¼ cup of the mixture onto griddle for each pancake. Turn when the edges of the pancakes begin to look dry and bubbles appear on the surface. Brown both sides.

GARLIC

Some people love the taste and smell of garlic; others hate it. But when it comes to health benefits, people on both sides of the issue can't argue with success or the research: *Allium sativum* has been highly effective in treating ailments ranging from infections to snake bites to high blood pressure. Sanskrit records show that it was used as a medicine about 5,000 years ago, and Chinese traditional medicine has embraced its healing power for more than 3,000 years. In 1858 Louis Pasteur wrote about its antibacterial properties, and garlic was used in both world wars to help prevent gangrene.

Today, garlic is very popular both as a food and a remedy. Most of the garlic grown in the United States comes from California.

Garlic Nutrition
Serving Size: 3 cloves (9 grams)
Calories: 13
Protein: 0.5 g
Total Fat: 0 g

Carbohydrates: 3 g
Fiber: 0.2 g
Cholesterol: 0 mg
Iron: 0.15 mg, 10% DRI

One to two cloves per day is suggested for maintaining health.

Health Benefits

Garlic contains a high concentration of sulfur-containing elements, including alliin, an amino acid that interacts with the enzyme alliinase when raw garlic is chewed or crushed. This interaction results in the formation of allicin, a substance believed to be responsible for many of garlic's health benefits.

- Several studies show that garlic can reduce cholesterol and triglyceride levels, which can help prevent atherosclerosis and other heart-related disease.
- Aged garlic extracts may prevent dementia by protecting neurons in the brain, and thus help fight cognitive decline and improve memory.
- Garlic can provide a modest but important decline in blood pressure.
- There is convincing evidence that garlic can help prevent cancer of the stomach and colon.
- Many studies provide evidence that garlic is effective against bacteria, viruses, fungi, and parasites, and has been effective in the treatment of infections, including bronchitis, the common cold, diarrhea, ear infections, urinary tract infections, and vaginitis.
- A substance called diallyl sulfide, found in garlic, appears to ward off carcinogens produced by meat and fish cooked at high temperatures. Researchers at Florida A&M University believe diallyl sulfide may help prevent certain forms of cancer.

How to Select and Store

Look for garlic that has firm, plump bulbs and with the roots still attached. Garlic that is sprouting (has a green

shoot) is often bitter. Store your garlic in a cool, dry place or
in the refrigerator.

RED GARLIC SOUP
Serves 2–3
3 lbs ripe tomatoes, peeled and chopped
4 garlic cloves, crushed
¼ cup red bell pepper, chopped
2 Tbs olive oil
1 Tbs white vinegar
1 Tbs balsamic vinegar
Salt and ground black pepper

Steam or sauté the chopped red bell pepper in a small amount
of water until tender. Puree the tomatoes in a food processor
with the garlic and olive oil. Strain the puree to remove the
tomato seeds or, if you prefer, leave them in. Stir in the vinegars, red peppers, and season with salt and pepper as desired.
Chill.

GARLIC SWEET POTATOES
Serves 4
1½ lbs sweet potatoes, cooked and quartered
2 garlic cloves, minced
2 Tbs olive oil
1 tsp cumin seed
½ tsp turmeric
3 Tbs fresh cilantro or parsley, minced

Heat 1 Tbs oil in a large skillet and sauté the garlic until soft.
Do not brown. Set aside. Heat the second Tbs of oil, add the
cumin seed and sauté until fragrant, about 1 minute. Add the
potatoes, turmeric, and garlic and sauté until the potatoes
are browned. Sprinkle with the parsley or cilantro.

GINGER

Ginger (*Zingiber officinale*) is a tropical plant whose under-ground stem (rhizome) is popular both for cooking and for its medicinal qualities. Since antiquity, ginger has been used as a medicine in Asian, Arabic, and Indian cultures to treat a range of conditions, including diarrhea, nausea, heart conditions, arthritis, and indigestion. Ginger is a native of Asia, and the world's largest producers of ginger are India and China.

Ginger Nutrition
  Serving Size: 1 Tbs, ground
  Calories: 19
  Protein: 0.5 g
  Total Fat: 0.3 g
  Carbohydrates: 3.8 g
  Fiber: 0.7 g
  Cholesterol: 0 mg

Health Benefits
  The health advantages of ginger don't lie in its vitamin and mineral content but in components called gingerols, which are unique to ginger.

- Several studies show that ginger helps reduce nausea and vomiting associated with pregnancy. Pregnant woman should take fresh rather than dried ginger root during pregnancy.
- Ginger may also be helpful in reducing symptoms of motion sickness (nausea, sweating, vomiting), although not all studies have had positive results.
- Several preliminary studies indicate that ginger may lower cholesterol and help prevent blood clots and ath-erosclerosis.
- When used as a tea, ginger can relieve symptoms of the common cold and flu, as well as menstrual cramps, headache, and sore throat.

- Gingerols appear to be responsible for relieving inflammation associated with arthritis and other inflammatory conditions.
- Ginger may be helpful in reducing inflammation associated with migraine, although more research is needed in this area.
- In lab studies, experts at the University of Minnesota found that gingerols can kill colorectal cancer cells, while researchers at the University of Michigan discovered these compounds are effective against ovarian cancer cells.

How to Select and Store

Head for the produce section when shopping for ginger: fresh ginger not only tastes better than the dried spice, but it has higher amounts of gingerol and other healthful ingredients. Fresh ginger should be firm and mold-free. Mature ginger is the most common type and it has a tough skin that you should peel before using; younger ginger is less available and does not need to be peeled.

Fresh, unpeeled ginger can be stored in the refrigerator, where it will stay fresh for up to three weeks, or in the freezer, where it will keep for up to six months. Ground ginger powder should be stored in a cool, dark place in a tightly closed glass container. It will stay fresh for about one year if stored in the refrigerator.

GINGERED BREAKFAST DRINK
Serves 1
½ cup orange juice
¼ cup unsweetened pineapple juice
½ ripe banana
½ tsp grated fresh ginger root
2 small ice cubes

Place all ingredients in a blender and process until smooth.

GINGER CARROT SOUP

Serves 4
2 Tbs olive oil
1 small onion, chopped
⅛ cup finely chopped ginger root
2 cloves garlic, minced
3½ cups vegetable broth
½ cup dry white wine
1 lb carrots, peeled and cut into ½" pieces
1 Tbs fresh lemon juice
Dash curry powder

In a large stock pot, sauté the onion, ginger, and garlic over medium heat for 15 minutes. Add the broth, wine, and carrots. Heat to boiling, reduce heat, and simmer uncovered for 40–45 minutes. Puree the soup in a blender or food processor. Season with lemon juice and curry powder. Serve hot or cold.

GRAPEFRUIT

Unlike many other fruits and vegetables, grapefruit do not have a long history. They were first discovered in the eighteenth century in Barbados and are believed to be the result of accidental cross breeding between the orange and the pomelo (also known as pummelo or shaddock). The name "grapefruit" was given to the fruit in 1814 because of the way the fruit hangs in clusters in the trees.

Grapefruit seeds were brought to Florida in 1823 by Count Odette Phillipe, and after years of resistance by the public, the thick-skinned citrus caught on and became a commercial crop in the late nineteenth century. Florida is the major producer of grapefruit in the United States, followed by California, Arizona, and Texas.

Grapefruit Nutrition
Serving Size for Both: 1 cup w/juice, all areas

Red and Pink Grapefruit
Calories: 97
Protein: 1.77 g
Total Fat: 0.3
Carbohydrates: 24.5 g
Fiber: 3.7 g
Cholesterol: 0 mg
Calcium: 51 mg, 5% DRI
Vitamin A: 2,645 IU, 102% DRI
Vitamin C: 72 mg, 87% DRI
Potassium: 310 mg, 7% DRI

White Grapefruit
Calories: 76
Protein: 1.59 g
Total Fat: 0.23 g
Carbohydrates: 19.3 g
Fiber: 2.5 g
Cholesterol: 0 mg
Calcium: 28 mg, 3% DRI
Vitamin A: 76 IU, 3% DRI
Vitamin C: 76.6 mg, 93% DRI
Potassium: 340 mg, 7% DRI

Health Benefits
You may think grapefruit provide the same health benefits as oranges, but there are some notable differences, even among grapefruit themselves. For example, red and pink grapefruit have more than thirty times the amount of vitamin A of white grapefruit, and they also have more fiber. Here is a rundown of the grapefruit's health advantages.

- Grapefruit stimulates the digestive system and can relieve heartburn, gas, and bloating.
- You don't need to eat grapefruit to reap its benefits: grapefruit juice applied to the skin can help treat oily

skin and acne. (Grapefruit should not be applied to broken skin.)

- Pink and red grapefruit contain lycopene, the phytonutrient that is associated with a reduced risk of prostate cancer and with the prevention and treatment of eye disorders, including cataracts, glaucoma, and macular degeneration.
- Pectin, found in grapefruit membranes and rind, helps reduce cholesterol.
- Red/pink grapefruit appears to be superior to white when it comes to lowering cholesterol and triglycerides. A Hebrew University study found that patients with high cholesterol who ate red grapefruit for 30 days lowered their total cholesterol by 15.5 percent while those who ate white grapefruit lowered their cholesterol by 7.6 percent. Triglycerides declined by 17.2 percent and 5.6 percent, respectively. Patients who did not eat grapefruit did not show any declines.
- Grapefruit contains phytonutrients called limonoids, which inhibit the development of tumors by promoting the formation of an enzyme involved in detoxification. Grapefruit pulp also contains glucarates, which may help prevent breast cancer.

How to Select and Store

The best grapefruit are heavy for their size, have relatively smooth, thin skin, and are firm yet mildly giving when you apply gentle pressure. Discolored or scratched skin does not affect the taste or quality of grapefruit. They should smell sweet at room temperature, but have little or no fragrance when they are cold. Grapefruit can be kept at room temperature if you plan to use them within a few days, or they can be refrigerated for two to three weeks.

BROILED GRAPEFRUIT
Serves 1–2
1 medium grapefruit

2 tsp honey
¼ tsp ground cinnamon

Cut the grapefruit in half and loosen each section. Place the grapefruit halves cut side up in a baking pan. Drizzle 1 tsp of honey on each half and sprinkle each with cinnamon. Broil 4 inches from the heat for 2–3 minutes until the fruit bubbles. Serve warm.

GRAPEFRUIT TURKEY SALAD
Serves 3–4
1 ½ cups grapefruit sections in bite-size pieces
2 cups cooked turkey or chicken, diced
¼ cup chopped celery
1 small red onion, minced
¼ cup low-fat mayonnaise
¼ cup low-fat plain yogurt
¼ cup fresh parsley, minced

Combine all ingredients and mix thoroughly. Serve on greens.

GRAPES

Grapes were one of the first fruits to be cultivated. Archaeologists have found fossil evidence of grapes in Iran that dates back 8,000 years. Of the thousands of varieties of grapes grown around the world, all can be classified as either American or European. American grapes have loose skin that slips off when you bite the fruit; European grapes have tighter skin. Both types are available either with or without seeds.

European grapes reached the United States in the late eighteenth century when Spanish missionaries brought them north from Mexico. Today California is the leading producer of table (for eating or making into raisins) and wine grapes. The grapes most Americans enjoy are red and green Thompson seedless table grapes.

Grape Nutrition
Serving Size: 1 cup red or green Thompson
Calories: 104
Protein: 1 g
Total Fat: 0.2 g
Carbohydrates: 27.3 g
Fiber: 1.4 g
Cholesterol: 0 mg
Vitamin C: 16.3 mg, 19% DRI

Health Benefits
Although grapes are not a rich source of many vitamins and minerals (except vitamin C), they really shine when it comes to phytonutrients, especially the polyphenols. Let's look at what grapes and grape juice have to offer.

- Grape skin contains the polyphenol resveratrol, which once in the body converts to an anticancer agent that destroys cancer cells.
- A *Journal of Nutrition* study shows that grapes may prevent the accumulation of plaque and the development of lesions in your arteries, thus helping prevent atherosclerosis, heart attack, stroke, and other cardiovascular conditions.
- Grapes also contain the polyphenol tannin, which scientists discovered can hinder or destroy viruses, including the HIV virus.
- The proanthocyanidins found in grape seeds (eat the seeds!) promote the destruction of cancer cells, including those responsible for skin cancer, according to a 2007 study published in *Experimental Dermatology*.
- Grape seeds also have the potential to reduce bad cholesterol levels and help prevent atherosclerosis, according to a 2007 study from Japan.
- Researchers find that purple grape juice is helpful in preventing the development of cardiovascular disease.

How to Select and Store

Look for grapes that are plump, tender, well formed, and firmly attached to their stems. At home, store them in a covered container or plastic bag in the refrigerator, where they should stay fresh for two to three days. Table grapes are crisp when chilled. Grapes can be frozen and make a tasty, cool snack right from the freezer.

WILD RICE AND GRAPE SALAD

Serves 8–10 side dishes
6 oz wild rice, cooked
8-oz can of sliced water chestnuts, drained
½ cup chopped celery
1 cup halved seedless red grapes
½ cup sliced green onions
3 Tbs olive oil
3 Tbs lemon juice
¼ tsp pepper
⅔ cup chopped walnuts

Cook the wild rice and put aside to cool. In a large bowl, combine the rice, water chestnuts, celery, green onions, and grapes. In a jar, combine the olive oil, lemon juice, and pepper. Shake well and pour over the rice mixture. Toss and chill for at least 4 hours. Before serving, mix in the walnuts.

GRAPE SALSA

1 medium orange, peeled and cut into small pieces
½ lb seedless red grapes, cut into quarters
½ cup chopped red bell pepper
¼ cup chopped cilantro
¼ cup chopped green onions
1 Tbs minced jalapenos
½ cup grape juice
1 Tbs fresh lime juice

Combine all ingredients in a large bowl and mix thoroughly. Serve with chips.

GREENS

"Leafy greens" is a phrase you often see when reading about health, and for good reason: these vegetables pack a tremendous amount of nutrients into their leaves. Greens is a broad category which for our purposes includes beet greens, mustard greens, kale, dandelion greens, collard greens, Swiss chard, and turnip greens. (We cover spinach and lettuce in separate entries.)

Collard greens were cultivated by the ancient Greeks and Romans, while mustard greens originated in the Himalayan region of India more than 5,000 years ago. Kale came from Asia Minor, and Swiss chard actually first grew in Sicily and got its Swiss name from the Swiss botanist who gave the vegetable its scientific name.

Greens Nutrition

Serving Size for all entries: 1 cup cooked, chopped

Mustard Greens

Calories: 21
Protein: 3.1 g
Total Fat: 0.3 g
Carbohydrates: 2.9 g
Fiber: 2.8 g
Cholesterol: 0 mg
Calcium: 104 mg, 10% DRI
Vitamin C: 35 mg, 43% DRI
Folate: 102 mcg, 26% DRI
Vitamin A: 8,852 IU, 340% DRI
Vitamin K: 419 mcg, 399% AI

Swiss Chard

Calories: 35
Protein: 3.3 g
Total Fat: 0.14 g
Carbohydrates: 7.2 g
Fiber: 3.7 g

Cholesterol: 0 mg
Calcium: 102 mg, 10% DRI
Iron: 3.95 mg, 30% DRI
Magnesium: 150 mg, 39% DRI
Vitamin C: 31 mg, 38% DRI
Vitamin A: 10,717 IU, 412% DRI
Vitamin K: 572 mcg, 543% AI

Kale

Calories: 36
Protein: 2.5 g
Total Fat: 0.5 g
Carbohydrates: 7.3 g
Fiber: 2.6 g
Cholesterol: 0 mg
Calcium: 94 mg, 9% DRI
Iron: 1.17 mg, 9% DRI
Vitamin C: 53 mg, 65% DRI
Vitamin A: 17,707 IU, 680% DRI
Vitamin K: 1,062 mcg, 1011% AI

Collard Greens

Calories: 49
Protein: 4 g
Total Fat: 0.7 g
Carbohydrates: 9.3 mg
Fiber: 5.3 mg
Cholesterol: 0 mg
Calcium: 266 mg, 27% DRI
Iron: 2.2 mg, 17% DRI
Vitamin C: 34 mg, 41% DRI
Folate: 177 mcg, 44% DRI
Vitamin A: 15,417 IU, 593% DRI
Vitamin K: 836 mcg, 796% AI

All of the greens have high levels of lutein, zeaxanthin, and beta-carotene, with kale having the highest levels of these phytonutrients.

Health Benefits

It's impossible to sing all the praises of all these greens, so we'll just give you a few to ponder. All of the greens have high levels of lutein, zeaxanthin, and beta-carotene, with kale having the highest levels of these phytonutrients. Here are some of the health benefits that spring from these leafy wonders.

- Both collard greens and kale are also members of the cruciferous family, along with broccoli and cauliflower. Therefore they also have cancer-prevention characteristics. Studies show that people who eat the most cruciferous vegetables have a much lower risk of prostate, colorectal, and lung cancers compared with people who eat other vegetables.
- The high levels of lutein, zeaxanthin, and beta-carotene in leafy greens help ward off serious eye diseases, including cataracts, glaucoma, and macular degeneration.
- All greens, but especially collards, are a very good plant source of calcium for bone health. This is important for people who shun dairy products.
- The abundant antioxidants in leafy greens are instrumental in boosting and maintaining immune system health, and thus may ward off infections, including the common cold, ear infections, flu, gingivitis, urinary tract infections, vaginitis, among others. The antioxidants also are anti-inflammatory agents, helping reduce symptoms of arthritis, asthma, bursitis, and fibromyalgia.
- The combination of calcium and magnesium found in leafy greens may reduce symptoms of menopause and PMS, including bloating, hot flashes, headache, cramping, and mood swings.
- The iron content of greens can help ward off and treat anemia.

How to Select and Store

Greens should be crisp and a vibrant color. Avoid greens that have yellow or dry leaves, or with stalks that are coarse or fibrous. Collards should be stored in the crisper section of the refrigerator or in a plastic bag with holes in it. They tend to last longer than do mustard greens, Swiss chard, or kale, all of which should be stored wrapped in plastic in the refrigerator, where they will keep for only a few days.

SPICY GREENS
Serves 4
3 cups kale
3 cups mustard greens
1 tsp olive oil
¼ tsp each: cumin seeds, mustard seeds, green
   chili peppers
¾ tsp salt
1 tsp garlic, minced
1 lime wedge
4 tsp water

Clean greens and cut the leaves into strips 1 inch by 4 inches. Steam in 4 tsp of water in a steamer pot until they are wilted, 5–10 minutes. Set aside. In a small saucepan, heat the oil and add the mustard seeds and cumin seeds until they sizzle. Add the green chili pepper, salt, and garlic, and sauté until lightly browned. Pour mixture over the greens. Season with lime.

COLLARDS AND BEANS
Serves 6
1 Tbs olive oil
2 cloves garlic, sliced
1 bunch collard greens, chopped
2 Tbs cider vinegar
½ cup water
1½ cups cooked kidney beans (canned is okay)
½ tsp hot pepper sauce to taste
Salt and pepper to taste

Sauté the garlic in a large pot over medium heat for about 1 minute; add the greens, vinegar, 2 Tbs water, and hot sauce.

Cook and stir often for about 5 minutes. Cover and cook 5 more minutes. Add the beans and remaining water. Cover and cook for 10 minutes. Stir in salt, pepper, and more hot sauce if desired.

GREEN TEA

Green tea, and tea in general, is a beverage with roots in ancient China. Legends about its origins abound: some say a Chinese emperor discovered the drink; Buddhists say Buddha has that honor; and the Chinese god of agriculture is also credited with its discovery.

Regardless of its origins, green tea has been enjoyed for its taste and medicinal value for about 5,000 years. In 350 AD, Chinese literature recorded how to brew green tea. Between 1405 and 1433, Chinese seamen depended on green tea to prevent scurvy, which killed many European sailors several years later. Today we know that it was the antioxidants in the tea that prevented the disease.

Green tea, as well as black and oolong varieties, come from the leaves of the *Camellia sinensis* plant. What distinguishes these teas from each other is how they are processed. Green tea is made by heating the leaves—usually by steaming—immediately after they are picked. This process prevents the fermentation that makes black and oolong tea. The leaves are then rolled and dried.

The world's leading tea producer is India, followed by China and Kenya. Tea is the second most consumed beverage in the world, bested only by water.

Green Tea Nutrition

Green tea has no calories and virtually zero percent of the nutrients usually listed in this space. However, green tea is rich in flavonoids, which make up thirty percent of the dry weight of green tea leaves. You can read about some of the benefits of the flavonoids below.

Health Benefits

The health benefits of green tea are due mainly to a type of flavonoid called catechins, the most potent of which is epigallocatechin gallate (EGCG). This antioxidant is about 25 to 100 times more potent than vitamins C and E. One cup of green tea has antioxidant effects greater than those from a serving of carrots, strawberries, or broccoli.

- EGCG appears to increase oxidation of fats, and can help reduce body fat and promote weight loss, according to a recent study published in the *Journal of the American College of Nutrition.*
- EGCG has been shown to inhibit the growth and spread of pancreatic and prostate cancer cells in several studies.
- Catechins may help lower the risk of cardiovascular disease by reducing the absorption of cholesterol, lowering blood pressure, and destroying free radicals.
- Green tea is effective in reducing the buildup of dental plaque, which helps prevent the development of gingivitis
- New research indicates that EGCG and the amino acid L-theanine found in green tea may help improve memory and learning. In one study, for example, elderly people who drank more than two cups a day of green tea reduced their odds of cognitive impairment by sixty-four percent.
- A large study found that, compared with people who drank less than one cup of green tea daily, those who drank five or more had a significantly lower risk of death from all causes, especially cardiovascular disease: women had a sixty-two percent lower risk and men had a forty-two percent lower risk of dying from stroke.
- Several studies indicate that the polyphenols in green tea protect dopamine neurons, which are involved in Parkinson's disease.

How to Select and Store

Many people are very serious about shopping for quality green tea, and there are many different types from which to choose. A general shopping tip if you are looking at loose green tea is to pinch a small amount between your fingers and smell it: it should smell slightly sweet and grassy. Green tea comes primarily from India, China, and Japan, and each region has its own special varieties. Organic green teas come mainly from India and California.

To store loose green tea or tea bags, use a ceramic or opaque glass container that has a tight lid. The container should be just large enough to accommodate the tea, as tea that is exposed to air continues to oxidize. Store the container in a cool, dry place; do not refrigerate.

GREEN TEA VEGGIES

Serves 4
2 Tbs olive oil
2 Tsp chopped fresh red chili pepper
1 tsp grated lemon peel
1 tsp loose tea leaves
4 cups broccoli florets
1 cup yellow or green squash, cut into ¼-inch slices
½ cup brewed green tea
¼ cup red bell pepper, chopped
Salt and pepper to taste

In a skillet or wok, stir-fry the chili pepper, lemon peel, and tea leaves in the oil for 1 minute. Add the broccoli and squash and stir-fry for 2 minutes. Add the brewed tea and bell pepper. Season with salt and pepper, and cook until most of the liquid evaporates.

GREEN TEA DIP

Makes 18 tablespoons
3 green tea bags
1 cup low-fat cream cheese or ricotta cheese

2 Tbs finely minced basil leaves
1 Tbs finely minced green tea leaves

Place the tea bags in 8 ounces of near-boiling water and allow
to steep for 3 to 5 minutes. Remove the tea bags and squeeze
out the liquid. Refrigerate if not using immediately. Place the
cheese, basil, and tea leaves in a blender and mix until smooth.
Gradually add the brewed tea until the mixture is spreadable.
Transfer the mixture to a covered container and refrigerate for
at least 1 hour.

GUAVA

Guava (*Psidium* spp) is a tropical and subtropical fruit that is
shaped like a pear, and has a green rind and pink flesh. Some describe the taste as being a cross between a pear and strawberries.

Guava originated in South and Central America, most
likely around Peru and Mexico. Little is known about its history, although it was mentioned in 1526 by Gonzalo Hernan-
dez de Oveido, who called the fruit "guayaba apple." He noted
that the fruit was grown throughout the West Indies and was
being cultivated by the Indians.

Guava thrives in a wide range of places around the world,
from India to Spain, Malaysia, Latin America, and New
Zealand. In the United States, California, Hawaii, and Florida
produce the fruit.

Guava Nutrition
Serving Size: 1 cup
Calories: 112
Protein: 4.2 g
Total Fat: 1.5 g
Carbohydrates: 23.6 g
Fiber: 8.9 g
Cholesterol: 0 mg
Vitamin A: 1,030 IU, 40% DRI
Vitamin C: 377 mg, 460% DRI

Vitamin B-6: 0.18 mg, 12% DRI
Potassium: 688 mg, 14% AI

Health Benefits

A guava has three times more vitamin C than an orange, high amounts of lycopene, and is an excellent source of fiber. To get the most out of your guava, do not peel it: the edible rind contains a very high amount of vitamin C. Here are some reasons to bite into a guava today.

- Lycopene has been shown to protect the eyes from development of cataracts, glaucoma, and macular degeneration.
- Preliminary evidence from several studies suggests that guava has anticancer properties.
- The very high vitamin C content of guava makes it a natural booster of the immune system and thus can help fight infections, including bronchitis, the common cold, flu, urinary tract infections, and vaginitis.
- Vitamin C is effective against symptoms of seasonal allergies.
- Guava contains an important fiber called pectin, which helps reduce cholesterol levels and assists in controlling blood sugar levels. Pectin can also work to maintain a healthy bowel and avoid diarrhea, diverticular disease, irritable bowel, and similar intestinal disorders.

How to Select and Store

Choose a guava that is not too green; it's okay to have some yellow skin and a few spots. The fruit should be tender and give to gentle pressure but not be mushy. Keep the fruit at room temperature until it is soft. Once it is ripe, it will keep for two days in the refrigerator if you put it in a plastic or paper bag.

GUAVA SALAD
Serves 2
1 guava, cut into chunks
1 banana, sliced

1 orange, in bite-size pieces
1 tsp lemon juice
1 Tbs mint leaves, chopped
3 Tbs chopped walnuts

Combine all ingredients and enjoy.

GUAVA SMOOTHIE
Serves 2–3
½ cup guava
½ cup banana
2 cups nonfat milk or nonfat vanilla soymilk
1 Tbs honey

Process all ingredients in a blender until smooth.

KEFIR

You can start your day—or give yourself a boost any time of the day—with a cup of pleasure. Kefir (ke´-fer), which loosely translated means "pleasure," is a fermented milk beverage that originated centuries ago in the Caucasus Mountains in the former Soviet Union. This tangy, naturally sweet drink contains probiotics, those friendly, healthful bacteria we talk about elsewhere in this book.

Kefir is highly regarded in Russia, Asia, and more recently Western Europe and the United States for its healing qualities. In Russia it is used to treat conditions ranging from atherosclerosis and allergies to gastrointestinal disorders and cancer. A growing number of scientific studies are discovering that kefir can boost the immune system and benefit the gastrointestinal system. Kefir is becoming increasingly more available in both natural and mainstream food stores in the United States.

Kefir Nutrition
Serving Size: 8 ounces, low-fat, plain (all information is from Lifeway brand)

Calories: 120
Protein: 14 g
Total Fat: 3 g
Carbohydrates: 12 g
Fiber: 3 g
Cholesterol: 10 mg
Vitamin A: 10% DRI
Vitamin D: 25% DRI
Calcium: 30% DRI

Health Benefits

One look at the nutritional panel on kefir, and you'll see that it is a great source of protein, calcium, and vitamin D, all critical not only for bone health but for many other essential functions as well. Kefir also provides vitamin B-1, B-12, and vitamin K. But it is the probiotics that make kefir unusual, as it is one of the few excellent food sources of these beneficial bacteria. In fact, kefir contains a greater and more diversified selection of beneficial bacteria than yogurt, plus it contains beneficial yeasts, which are not found in yogurt. Let's look at how kefir may improve your health.

- A study published in *Immunobiology* reports that kefir has anti-inflammatory and anti-allergy qualities, and may be useful in the prevention and treatment of asthma and eczema.
- Kefir provides probiotics that have proven effective in preventing and treating gastrointestinal conditions, including diarrhea, diverticular disease, irritable bowel syndrome, and ulcers.
- Urinary tract infections and vaginitis can be successfully prevented and treated with probiotics.
- Including kefir in your diet may reduce your risk for colorectal cancer, as the probiotics help maintain a healthy balance of bacteria in the intestinal tract.
- Tooth and gum disorders, including gingivitis, can be prevented and treated by including probiotics in your diet.

- Probiotics may help reduce several risk factors for cardiovascular disease, including inflammation and high LDL cholesterol levels.
- Probiotics may reduce the duration and severity of cold and flu symptoms, according to several studies. One study also found that the incidence of respiratory tract infections (e.g., cold, flu) was thirteen percent lower in people who had consumed probiotics than people who had not.

How to Select and Store

Kefir is available in health food stores, but increasingly it can be found in mainstream grocery stores in the dairy section. It typically contains more than two dozen strains of beneficial bacteria and yeasts. Always check the "Sell By" date on the container and store the kefir in the refrigerator. Nonfat, low-fat, and regular varieties are available, as are plain, vanilla, and fruit flavors. You can also make your own kefir at home using kefir starting culture, which is available online and from many natural health food stores.

KEFIR SALAD DRESSING
Makes 2 cups
2 cups fresh plain nonfat or low-fat kefir
1 Tbs fresh parsley, chopped
1 Tbs fresh lemon zest, chopped
1 Tbs flaxseed oil
1 Tbs fresh garlic, minced
1 tsp salt
½ tsp xanthan gum

Combine all ingredients except the xanthan gum and blend. Slowly add xanthan gum and continue to stir until the dressing thickens. Refrigerate for 6–8 hours to allow the dressing to attain full flavor.

CHOCOLATE BANANA KEFIR
Serves 1
6 oz nonfat or low-fat kefir, plain
½ oz dark chocolate, shaved
½ banana
1 Tbs honey

Combine all ingredients in a blender and process until smooth.

LEMONS AND LIMES

Lemons are the result of cross breeding between the lime and the citron, and are believed to have originated in India or China. The yellow fruit found its way to Europe in the eleventh century, and was brought to the Americans by Christopher Columbus in 1493. Florida, the main lemon producer in the United States, has been growing the fruit since the sixteenth century. Today, the major producers of lemons are the United States, Italy, Spain, Greece, and Israel.

Limes have a similar history. They originated in Southeast Asia and were introduced into Northern Africa around the tenth century. The green citrus arrived in Spain in the thirteenth century and crossed the Atlantic with Columbus in 1493. Like lemons, limes were first grown in Florida beginning in the sixteenth century. The leading commercial producers of limes today are Brazil, Mexico, and the United States.

The main claim to fame for lemons and limes is their high vitamin C content, which saved many people from developing scurvy in the eighteenth and nineteenth centuries. Although most people don't sink their teeth into these citrus, they do use them to enhance the flavor of many other foods.

Lemon Nutrition
Serving Size: ¼ cup juice
Calories: 15
Protein: 0.2 g
Total Fat: 0 g

Carbohydrates: 5.2 g
Fiber: 0.3
Cholesterol: 0 mg
Vitamin C: 28 mg, 34% DRI

Lime Nutrition

Serving Size: ¼ cup juice
Calories: 16
Protein: 0.2 g
Total Fat: 0 g
Carbohydrates: 5 g
Fiber: 0.2 g
Cholesterol: 0 mg
Vitamin C: 18 mg, 22% DRI

Health Benefits

Both lemons and limes contain special flavonoids and good levels of vitamin C. What do these mean for your health?

- Limes contain flavonol glycosides, which studies show can interfere with cancer cell growth and act as an antibiotic.
- Substances called limonoids, also found in lemons and limes, may fight various cancers, including mouth, skin, lung, breast, stomach, and colon cancer.
- The vitamin C content of lemons and limes can help boost and strengthen the immune system, and guard against conditions such as bronchitis, the common cold, ear infections, fever, flu, and hives.

How to Select and Store

Thin is in when it comes to picking lemons: good-quality lemons have thin rather than thick peels. The fruit should be heavy for its size and have a fine-grained texture. Lemons usually stay fresh at room temperature for one week if you keep them out of the sun. If you refrigerate lemons, they should last up to four weeks.

When choosing limes, look for fruit that is firm and heavy

for its size. The skin should be glossy; limes are more tart when they are deep green and turn more yellow as they ripen. Limes kept at room temperature should remain fresh for up to one week if they are not exposed to sunlight. In the refrigerator, limes should be wrapped in a loosely sealed plastic bag and will keep for up to two weeks.

If you need just a few drops of lemon or lime juice, pierce the skin with a toothpick and squeeze out what you need, then reinsert the toothpick, put the fruit into a plastic bag, and refrigerate.

LEMON SMOOTHIE
Serving Size: 2 cups plus
1 cup plain yogurt
¾ cup lemonade
½ cup crushed pineapple
1 banana
Ice

Place all the ingredients in a blender and blend until frothy.

LIME DRESSING
Makes about ½ cup dressing
¼ cup olive oil
1 tsp lime zest
¼ cup lime juice
2 Tbs chopped cilantro
1 Tbs water
1 clove garlic, minced
¼ tsp each: salt, ground cumin, ground cardamom

Combine all ingredients in a shaker bottle and shake well.

LENTILS

Lentils are a tiny, highly nutritious member of the legume family. Experts have determined that lentils are one of the first foods to be cultivated; seeds dating about 8,000 years have been found at archaeological sites in the Middle East.

Today, lentils are a traditional favorite in many countries, including India and throughout the Middle East, and Italy, where people have a custom of eating lentils on New Year's Eve or New Year's Day with the hope that they will be financially secure during the rest of the year. They are also a staple food during Lent.

Lentil Nutrition

Serving Size: 1 cup cooked
Calories: 230
Protein: 17.8 g
Total Fat: 0.75 g
Carbohydrates: 40 g
Fiber: 15.6 g
Cholesterol: 0 mg
Folate: 358 mcg, 89% DRI
Iron: 6.6 mg, 51% DRI
Phosphorus: 356 mg, 50% DRI
Zinc: 2.5 mg, 28% DRI

Health Benefits

Lentils are known for their high fiber, protein, and mineral content while being virtually fat-free.

• Lentils contain high levels of both soluble and insoluble fiber, which helps keep you regular and also helps prevent colorectal cancer, constipation, diabetes, diarrhea, diverticular disease, heart disease, hemorrhoids, high cholesterol, irritable bowel, and stroke.
• A high-fiber diet can also help prevent heart disease. Research published in the *Archives of Internal Medicine* shows that people who ate the most water-soluble fiber had a fifteen percent reduction in risk of coronary heart disease.
• The high levels of folate and magnesium in lentils can help prevent heart attack and enhance heart health: fo-

late helps reduce levels of homocysteine, while magnesium allows blood vessels to relax, which improves blood flow.

• People with anemia or chronic fatigue may benefit from eating lentils, as one cup contains fifty percent of the daily need for iron. This vital mineral plays a key role in energy production and metabolism.

How to Select and Store

Lentils are usually available in prepackaged containers and bulk bins. Any lentils you buy should be whole (not cracked) and moisture-free. If you prefer canned lentils, look for brands that do not contain salt or preservatives.

Dry lentils should be stored in an airtight container and kept in a cool, dark, dry place. Properly stored lentils usually keep for twelve months. Once lentils are cooked, they will keep fresh in the refrigerator for about three days if stored in a covered container.

LENTIL APRICOT SOUP

Serves 6–8

2 cups dry lentils
6 cups water
½ cup dried apricots, chopped
1½ cups onions, chopped
1 cup chopped green bell pepper
1 28-oz can crushed tomatoes
1 tsp allspice, ground
¼ tsp cinnamon, ground
¼ tsp cayenne

In a large pot, bring the water to a boil and add the lentils. Once the water begins to boil again, reduce the heat, cover, and cook the lentils until they begin to soften, about 10 minutes. Add all the remaining ingredients and simmer, stirring occasionally, until the vegetables are soft. Add more water if needed.

LENTIL-TOMATO-FETA SALAD
Serves 4 (side dish)
3 Tbs virgin olive oil
2 Tbs white wine vinegar
¼ tsp dried thyme
¼ cup sun-dried tomatoes packed in oil, chopped
1 cup lentils
3 cups water
½ cup feta cheese, crumbled

In a saucepan, bring salted water to a boil and add lentils. Cook until tender, about 20 minutes. In the meantime, combine the remaining ingredients except the feta in a bowl and whisk together. Drain the lentils and rinse gently. Place lentils in a bowl, add dressing, and gently stir in the feta.

LETTUCE

Oddly enough, the iceberg, red leaf, romaine, or butterhead lettuce in your salad bowl is a member of the sunflower family. Lettuce may also be the first vegetable memorialized with a statue: Emperor Caesar Augustus erected a monument to lettuce because he said the vegetable cured him of an illness.

Lettuce made its way to America from England in the 1600s in seed packets carried by John Winthrop, Jr. Today lettuce is the second most popular fresh vegetable in the United States, and Americans eat an average of thirty pounds of the greens each year. Most lettuce in the United States is grown in California and Arizona, but New Jersey, New York, New Mexico, and Colorado also make substantial contributions.

Lettuce Nutrition
Serving Size: all are 1 cup, shredded

Romaine
Calories: 8
Protein: 0.6 g

Total Fat: 0.1 g
Carbohydrates: 1.6 g
Fiber: 1.0 g
Cholesterol: 0 mg
Folate: 64 mcg, 16% DRI
Vitamin A: 2729 IU, 105% DRI
Vitamin K: 48 mcg, 45% AI
Manganese: 0.73 mg, 36% AI

Iceberg
Calories: 10
Protein: 0.6 g
Total Fat: 0.1 g
Carbohydrates: 2.1 g
Fiber: 0.9 g
Cholesterol: 0 mg
Folate: 21 mcg, 5% DRI

Green Leaf
Calories: 5
Protein: 0.5 g
Total Fat: 0 g
Carbohydrates: 1 g
Fiber: 0.5 g
Cholesterol: 0 mg
Folate: 14 mcg, 7% DRI
Vitamin A: 2666 IU, 100% DRI
Vitamin K: 62.5 mcg, 60% DRI

Health Benefits
Two nutritional nuggets to remember about lettuce is that the darker green leaves contain more nutrients than the lighter ones, and that iceberg is the least nutritious of the lettuce varieties. When it's salad time, explore beyond iceberg!

- Lettuce is an important source of vitamin K, which is essential for bone health. Studies show that low intake

of vitamin K is associated with an increased risk of
hip fracture in women.

- Low in calories, high in water content, and a good
  source of essential nutrients: lettuce is a great food to
  help fight obesity.
- Folate is heart-healthy because it helps keep homocysteine levels down and thus reduce the risk of heart attack and stroke.
- Vitamin A/beta-carotene is a heart-healthy nutrient as
  well, and it also helps prevent cataracts, glaucoma,
  and macular degeneration.
- Conditions that affect the skin and/or mucous membranes can benefit from vitamin A, including acne,
  canker sores, eczema, gingivitis, and psoriasis.

How to Select and Store

Regardless of the variety of lettuce you buy, the leaves
should be crisp and not wilted, brown, or yellow. If the lettuce
has a stem end, it should not be too brown.

Leaf and Romaine lettuce should be washed and dried before
you place it in a plastic bag or damp cloth and refrigerate it.
Boston and iceberg lettuce should not be washed before refrigerating. Romaine lettuce will keep for five to seven days; Boston
and leaf lettuce for two to three days. Do not store lettuce near
fruit that produces ethylene, such as bananas, pears, and apples,
as they will cause the lettuce to turn brown.

LETTUCE SOUP

Serves 4
2 small red or brown onions, finely chopped
1 small head Romaine lettuce, broken into small pieces
2 small red potatoes, peeled and chopped
3 cups water
2 Tbs olive oil
Salt and pepper to taste

Place all ingredients into a soup pot, bring to a boil, reduce
heat and simmer until all ingredients are soft. Season to taste.

GREEK LETTUCE WRAPS
Serves 2–3
2 large tomatoes, chopped
1 cucumber, chopped
½ green bell pepper, chopped
2 Tbs olive oil
⅓ cup black olive halves
1 green onion, chopped
½ cup crumbled feta cheese
6 butter lettuce leaves

Combine all ingredients except the lettuce leaves. Toss until blended. Chill or use at room temperature. Place some of the filling on each lettuce leaf, roll up, and enjoy.

LIMA BEANS

Children typically turn up their nose when lima beans are put on their plate, but adults often come to appreciate how tasty and nutritious these beans are. The most popular lima bean variety in the United States is the Fordhook or butterbean, but there are many others. Although lima beans are usually green or cream in color, certain varieties are red, purple, black or brown. All have a potato-like, slightly buttery texture. Sounds good!

Experts believe lima beans originated more than 7,000 years ago in Peru or Guatemala, and were carried around the world by Spanish and Portuguese explorers. Lima beans were introduced to the United States in the nineteenth century, and today most US commercial production is in California.

Lima Bean Nutrition
Serving Size: 1 cup, cooked
Calories: 216
Protein: 14.7 g
Total Fat: 0.7 g
Carbohydrates: 39 g

Fiber: 13 g
Cholesterol: 0 mg
Folate: 156 mcg; 39% DRI
Iron: 4.5 mg, 34% DRI
Molybdenum: 140 mcg, 311% DRI

Health Benefits

Lima beans are an excellent source of fiber, but they also have some other advantages up their pods. Let's look at a few of them.

- One cup of lima beans contains more than three times the DRI for molybdenum, an important trace mineral that detoxifies sulfites, a type of preservative found in many foods. People who have a bad reaction to sulfites (e.g., headache, rapid heartbeat, disorientation) frequently have low levels of molybdenum.
- That same cup of lima beans contains one-third of the DRI for iron. This mineral can help prevent and treat anemia and fatigue, especially in menstruating women who are at higher risk for iron deficiency. Children, adolescents, pregnant women, and nursing women also have a greater need for iron.
- Lima beans are an excellent source of soluble fiber and they are a good choice for people who have diabetes because they help control the rise in blood glucose (sugar) levels.
- The high fiber in lima beans also helps remove cholesterol from the body, which is key in the prevention of atherosclerosis, diabetes, high blood pressure, heart disease, and stroke.
- Fiber helps to maintain regularity and to prevent and treat constipation, diarrhea, diverticular disease, hemorrhoids, irritable bowel syndrome, and varicose veins.

How to Select and Store

You are much more likely to find dried than fresh lima beans in the market. Dried lima beans are available in prepackaged containers and bulk bins. Look for beans that are whole and without evidence of cracks or moisture. If you find fresh whole lima beans, choose beans that are firm, dark green, and glossy. If they are shelled, select beans that have green or greenish-white skins.

Store dried lima beans in an airtight container in a cool, dry, dark place, and they should keep fresh for up to six months. Once cooked, lima beans last only one day, even if you put them in a covered container in the refrigerator. If you don't plan to eat cooked lima beans within twenty-four hours, freeze them in a tightly sealed plastic bag. If you buy fresh lima beans, store them whole in the refrigerator, where they should stay fresh for two to three days.

LIMA BEAN CAKES
Makes 4–6 cakes
1 ½ cups lima beans, cooked and mashed
1 cup soft breadcrumbs
½ cup finely chopped onion
2 Tbs chopped parsley
1 tsp salt
¼ tsp pepper
2 Tbs olive oil

Combine the mashed beans, breadcrumbs, onion, parsley, salt, and pepper. Shape the mixture into small flat cakes. Refrigerate the cakes for 1 hour. In a large skillet, brown the cakes in olive oil, about 3 minutes per side.

LIMA BEAN SOUP
Makes 4 cups
2 15-oz cans of lima beans (butter beans)
¾ cup finely chopped carrots
1 ⅓ cups finely chopped celery
1 cup chopped tomatoes
6 cups water
2 Tbs margarine
½ cup finely chopped onion

2 Tbs chopped fresh coriander
2 Tbs flour
½ tsp salt

In a large saucepan, combine the carrots, celery, tomatoes, and water and bring to a boil. Reduce heat and simmer partially covered until the beans and vegetables are tender. In a small skillet, melt the margarine and sauté the onion and coriander for about 5 minutes. Stir in flour and cook for 1 minute. Add the lima beans to the large saucepan, stir well, and then stir in the onion/flour mixture. Simmer until the soup is slightly thickened, about 5 minutes. Season with salt.

MANGOES

For about 4,000 years, mangoes have been enjoyed by people of many cultures. Mangoes are believed to have originated in the foothills of the Himalayas. These original wild mangoes were much smaller than the modern, cultivated varieties, and they also had a turpentine-like taste, completely unlike the succulent fruit of today. Mangoes were carried to the Middle East and Africa by Persian traders, and then other traders brought the fruit to the West Indies and Brazil. Mangoes reached Florida in the 1830s and California in the 1880s.

More than 1,000 varieties of mangoes are grown around the world, and the ones enjoyed in the United States typically come from Mexico, the Caribbean, Haiti, and South America. Although India is the largest mango producer in the world, it exports very few because the fruit is so loved by its people.

Mango Nutrition
Serving Size: 1 cup slices
Calories: 107
Protein: 0.8 g
Total Fat: 0.5 g
Carbohydrates: 28 g

Fiber: 3 g
Cholesterol: 0 mg
Vitamin C: 46 mg, 56% DRI

Health Benefits

For many people, mangoes are a "foreign" fruit and not on their menu, and that's too bad because they offer several important nutrients, including fiber, and a change from ordinary fruit fare.

- Mangoes contain an enzyme, similar to the ones found in papayas and pineapple, that can aid digestion and heartburn.
- Mangoes contain many polyphenols, including quercetin, astragalin, gallic acid, and fisetin, that have potent antioxidant and anticancer properties.
- The potassium and magnesium in mangoes can help relieve heart problems, stress, and muscle cramps.
- The high fiber content in just one mango can help prevent constipation, diarrhea, diverticular disease, hemorrhoids, hypertension, and irritable bowel syndrome.
- Mangoes contain a significant amount of beta-carotene, which may help prevent and/or treat acne, bursitis, cataracts, the common cold, ear infections, eczema, gingivitis, herpes, macular degeneration, psoriasis, and urinary tract infections.

How to Select and Store

When shopping for mangoes, smell and squeeze. Ripe mangoes have a hearty, fruity aroma that you can smell at the stem end. Mangoes are ready to eat when they yield to gentle pressure and the skin has a yellow tinge, although they are also tasty when the skin is red, green, orange, or any combination. Mangoes can ripen at room temperature on a counter, or you can speed up the process by placing the fruit in a paper bag overnight. Once ripe, a mango can be refrigerated but should be eaten within two to three days.

MANGO MELON SOUP
Serves 6–8
3 mangoes, peeled and cubed
1 small cantaloupe, peeled and cubed
1 ripe banana, peeled and chunked
1 Tbs fresh lemon juice
Dash vanilla extract
Mint leaves for garnish

Place cantaloupe, banana, ½ of the mango cubes, lemon juice, and vanilla extract in a blender and process until smooth. Refrigerate the mixture for several hours or overnight. Refrigerate the remaining mango cubes separately. When you are ready to serve the soup, place the mango cubes in individual bowls and pour the mixture over the cubes. Garnish with mint leaves if desired.

MANGO SALSA
Makes about 3½ cups
1 mango, peeled, seeded and diced
1 avocado, peeled, pitted, and diced
4 medium tomatoes, diced
1 jalapeno pepper, seeded and minced
½ cup chopped fresh cilantro
3 cloves garlic, minced
1 tsp salt
2 Tbs fresh lime juice
¼ cup chopped red onion
2 Tbs olive oil

Combine all ingredients, stir thoroughly, and chill for about 30 minutes before serving.

MUSHROOMS

Many people think mushrooms are a vegetable, but they are actually a fungus, a "plant" that has no leaves, roots, flowers, or seeds. Even without all these features, mushrooms have long been regarded as having special powers. Forget Kryptonite: Superman might have done just fine if he had eaten mushrooms, if he believed in the folklore of Russia, Mexico, and China, which says that mushrooms give people superhuman strength.

Although there are dozens of varieties of mushrooms, button mushrooms—including white buttons and brown, or crimini—are among the most widely grown and consumed. Other popular varieties include portabellas, shiitaki, straw, and reishi mushrooms. The United States is a leading producer of button mushrooms, and Pennsylvania produces most of them.

Mushroom Nutrition

Serving Size: 1 cup, sliced, raw—brown/crimini button
Calories: 19
Protein: 1.8 g
Total Fat: 0 g
Carbohydrates: 3 g
Fiber: 0.4 g
Cholesterol: 0 mg
Copper: 0.3 mg, 33% DRI
Niacin, 2.7 mg, 18% DRI
Riboflavin: 0.4 mg, 33% DRI
Selenium: 18.7 mg, 33% DRI

Health Benefits

Mushrooms are a good source of most of the B vitamins, selenium, copper, and potassium, and they're low in calories as well. Although they are not vegetables, mushrooms should be a regular part of your fruit and vegetable intake.

- One cup of mushrooms provides one-third of the DRI for selenium, a mineral that may help decrease the risk of prostate cancer. The Baltimore Longitudinal Study on Aging, for example, found that men with the lowest selenium levels were four to five times more likely to develop prostate cancer than men who had the highest selenium levels.

- Selenium may assist in the treatment of allergies, atherosclerosis, cataracts, HIV/AIDS, and macular degeneration.
- One-third of the DRI for riboflavin can be found in just one three-ounce portabella mushroom cap. Riboflavin is important in the prevention of cataracts and in the formation of red blood cells.
- The copper in mushrooms may help reduce the symptoms of rheumatoid arthritis and in helping fight free-radical damage.
- Niacin is associated with memory loss and other cognitive functions. A Chicago study found that older adults who got the most niacin (22 mg daily) were 70 percent less likely to develop Alzheimer's disease than those who consumed the least amount (13 mg daily) of niacin.
- Mushrooms contain beta-glucan, a substance that can boost the immune system and offer anticancer benefits, including reduced tumor growth.

How to Select and Store

Regardless of the type of mushroom you choose, look for firm, unblemished caps that are free of mold and moisture, but are not dry. Refrigerate mushrooms in a paper—not plastic—bag that is loosely closed so the mushrooms do not get moist and spoil. Properly stored, fresh mushrooms should stay fresh for five days or longer. Do not wash mushrooms until just before you want to use them. Clean mushrooms by wiping them with a damp cloth or soft brush, or running them under cold water.

BAKED PORTABELLAS
Serves 4
4 large Portabella caps
1 cup olive oil
1 cup red wine vinegar
2 Tbs soy sauce
1 Tbs sugar
1 Tbs dried herbs
½ cup finely chopped fresh herbs

Combine all ingredients except the mushroom caps, whisk well, and let the marinade sit for one hour until the herbs soften. Slice the stems off the caps. Place the mushroom caps in a shallow dish and pour the marinade over them. Let the mushrooms marinate for 10 minutes, turning occasionally. Remove the mushrooms from the marinade, place on a baking tray and bake in a 350 F oven for 5–7 minutes. Serve immediately.

MUSHROOM CHILI
Serves 4
2 Tbs olive oil
3 cups white or brown button mushrooms, sliced
1 clove garlic
2 Tbs chili powder
1¼ cup vegetable broth
3 cups stewed tomatoes
1 15-oz can kidney beans
1 cup corn kernels

In a large saucepan, heat the oil, add the mushrooms and garlic, and cook until the mushrooms are tender and the liquid evaporates, about 5 minutes. Stir often. Stir in the chili powder and cook for 1 minute. Add the broth, stewed tomatoes, kidney beans, and corn. Bring to a boil, reduce heat, and simmer for 10 minutes.

OATS

The hearty oat has been cultivated for about two thousand years. Modern oats have their roots in a wild red oat that originated in Asia. Oats are most often used in two forms: as oatmeal and oat bran. Oatmeal is popular as a cereal and for baking; oat bran is the outermost layer of the oat kernel and is used in ways similar to wheat germ.

Oats were recognized for their healing properties even before they were used as food, and today they are appreciated for both purposes throughout Europe, Russia, and North

America. The major commercial producers of oats today are
Russia, the United States, Germany, Poland, and Finland.

Oatmeal Nutrition

Serving Size: 1 cup cooked, rolled or regular
Calories: 145
Protein: 6 g
Total Fat: 2 g
Carbohydrates: 25 g
Fiber: 4 g
Cholesterol: 0 mg
Manganese: 1.37 mg, 68.5% DRI
Selenium: 19 mcg, 34% DRI
Thiamin: 0.26 mg, 21% DRI

Oat Bran Nutrition

Serving Size: ¼ cup, uncooked
Calories: 58
Protein: 4 g
Total Fat: 1.6 g
Carbohydrates: 15.4 g
Fiber: 3.6 g
Cholesterol: 0 mg
Thiamin: 0.28 mg, 24% DRI
Magnesium: 55 mg, 14% DRI
Iron: 0.63 mg, 38% DRI

Health Benefits

Oatmeal does more than stick to your ribs and taste great
on a cold winter morning; it offers a host of health benefits
that can help *you* stick around longer. Here are a few of them.

• Oats, oatmeal, and oat bran contain beta-glucan, a type
of fiber that is especially effective at reducing cholesterol levels. Lower cholesterol levels can significantly
reduce the risk of stroke and heart disease. A study in
the *Archives of Internal Medicine* found that adults
who ate the most fiber (twenty-one grams daily) had

twelve percent less coronary heart disease and eleven percent less cardiovascular disease compared with people who ate five grams daily.

- Beta-glucan also significantly improves the immune system's response to bacterial infections, which may include bronchitis, ear infections, gingivitis, and urinary tract infections.
- Beta-glucan has the ability to reduce blood sugar levels, which is helpful for people at risk for or who have diabetes.
- Plant lignans are abundant in oats, and one special lignan called enterolactone is believed to protect against hormone-dependent cancers (e.g., breast, cervical, ovarian) and heart disease.
- Studies show that intake of whole grains and fish may reduce the risk of asthma in children by fifty percent. This response may be related to the omega-3 fatty acids in these foods.

How to Select and Store

Whether you buy oats in prepackaged containers or from a bulk bin, be sure they are moisture-free. Buy small quantities of oats at one time—about two months' worth—as oats can go rancid if kept for a long time. Store oatmeal and oat bran in an airtight container in a dry, cool, dark place and they should stay fresh for about two months.

OATMEAL SOUP
Serves 4
2 Tbs olive oil
1 onion, finely chopped
1 cup celery, chopped
½ cup uncooked steel-cut oats and 1 cup cooked oats
6 cups vegetable broth
3 Tbs parsley, chopped

In a large skillet, sauté the onion and celery until soft, about 5 minutes. Add the uncooked oatmeal and cook over medium-high heat, stirring constantly until the oatmeal is golden, about 3 minutes. Stir in the broth; add salt and pepper to taste. Bring to simmer and add cooked oatmeal, stir well, and simmer 5 minutes. Add parsley and serve.

CHOCOLATE OATMEAL
Makes 4½-cup servings
¼ cup chopped, pitted dates
1 cup old-fashioned rolled oats
2 Tbs flaked dark chocolate
Pinch of salt
2 cups water

Bring the water and salt to a boil and stir in the oats. Reduce the heat and simmer for about 10 minutes, stirring occasionally. Add the dates and chocolate, stir well, and continue cooking for another 2 to 3 minutes or until creamy as desired.

OLIVE OIL

Olive oil is the natural product of one of the oldest foods known to humankind. Olive trees originated in Crete about 7,000 years ago, and the fruits were enjoyed by people in various civilizations for several thousand years before they began to use the oil as a separate food item. Missionaries brought olives to California in the late eighteenth century.

Olive oil has long been on the menus of people living in Mediterranean countries, and in the past few decades it has become increasingly popular in the United States as a growing number of studies reveal its medicinal powers. Much of the olive oil consumed in the United States comes from Spain, Italy, Greece, Portugal, and Turkey.

Olive Oil Nutrition
Serving Size: 1 tablespoon
Calories: 119
Protein: 0 g

Total Fat: 13.5 g
  Monounsaturated Fat: 9.9 g
  Saturated Fat: 1.8 g
Carbohydrates: 0 g
Fiber: 0 g
Cholesterol: 0 mg

Health Benefits

When you look at the standard nutritional label on olive oil, you may wonder why it is always being touted as a healthful food. Except for fat, what's so great about olive oil? Scientists have discovered that not only is the fat beneficial, but olive oil also contains many "hidden" treasures. Note that extra virgin olive oil provides a greater amount of phytonutrients than refined olive oil. Let's start with the fat.

- A large study showed that exclusive use of olive oil resulted in a forty-seven percent reduced risk of coronary heart disease. One reason for this benefit is the high content of monounsaturated fat, which helps reduce cholesterol levels and thus helps prevent atherosclerosis. Another is the presence of phytonutrients called oleuropein, which helps prevent plaque from adhering to blood vessel walls.
- At least four studies found other substances in olive oil (beyond monounsaturated fat) that benefit the heart. These include antioxidants such as vitamin E, chlorophyll, carotenoids, and the polyphenol compounds tyrosol, oleuropein, and hydrotyrosol.
- People with diabetes who consume olive oil may have better insulin sensitivity, according to a 2007 study in *Diabetes Care.*
- Oleic acid, the main monounsaturated fatty acid in olive oil, can reduce the impact of a factor that is associated with aggressive growth of breast cancer tumors. This relationship was uncovered during a study conducted at Northwestern University in Chicago.

- The anti-inflammatory powers of monounsaturated fats are associated with lower rates of asthma and rheumatoid arthritis.
- Studies in both animals and people indicate that olive oil contains polyphenols that can interfere with or destroy the bacteria responsible for gastric ulcers— *Helicobacter pylori*. Olive oil greatly reduced ulcer size and significantly improved ulcer healing.

How To Select and Store

When shopping for olive oil, consider how you are going to use it. If you want to cook with it as well as drizzle it on prepared foods, then you need two different types of oil. An oil labeled "pure olive oil," "cooking grade olive oil," or just "olive oil" is fine for cooking. For prepared foods, look for virgin or extra-virgin oils.

Air, light, and heat will cause olive oil to turn rancid, so store olive oil in a dark area where the temperature remains fairly constant. The ideal temperature for storing olive oil is 57 degrees Fahrenheit, but 70 degrees Fahrenheit is acceptable. Refrigerating olive oil is not recommended if you have an expensive extra-virgin variety because condensation may develop and affect the flavor. Lesser grades of olive oil refrigerate well; although they will turn cloudy and may congeal, they will return to liquid once they warm up and the flavor should not be affected. Olive oil should be stored in tinted glass, porcelain, or stainless steel containers, never plastic or reactive metals (e.g. aluminum).

OLIVE OIL/ALMOND DRESSING

Makes ¾ cup
½ cup slivered blanched almonds
¼ cup olive oil
2 Tbs lime juice
2 Tbs water
½ tsp salt
¼ tsp ground black pepper

In a 350° F oven, bake the almonds on a baking sheet for about 5 minutes. Allow them to cool. Place all ingredients into a blender and process until smooth.

TIPS ON INCLUDING OLIVE OIL IN YOUR DIET

- Add a tablespoon to a glass of vegetable juice and shake well.
- Drizzle olive oil on steamed vegetables
- Mix olive oil with some of your favorite herbs, shake well, and use as a dipping oil for raw vegetables or bite-size pieces of whole-grain bread
- Instead of using red or white sauce on your pasta, drizzle olive oil and season with herbs and grated cheese.
- Whisk a tablespoon of olive oil into your pasta sauce
- Use olive oil instead of butter in some recipes. For example, olive oil can replace butter in mashed potatoes, casseroles, and pureed vegetables.

ONIONS

If you shed a few tears when you cut your next onion, be assured that the substances causing those tears also carry significant health benefits. Some of those advantages were recognized by ancient peoples, and today's researchers are now documenting them. They have quite a task ahead of them, as there are approximately 150 phytonutrients in onions.

Onions are believed to have originated in Central Asia, although some experts dispute this claim. Ancient Egyptians highly revered onions for their spiritual value and believed they represented eternal life, which is why onions were buried with the pharaohs.

Onion Nutrition
Serving Size: 1 cup chopped, raw
Calories: 64
Protein: 1.7 g

Total Fat: 0 g
Carbohydrates: 15 g
Fiber: 2.7 g
Cholesterol: 0 mg
Vitamin C: 12 mg, 14% DRI
Vitamin B-6: 0.19 mg, 13% DRI

Health Benefits

Scientists have identified approximately 150 phytonutrients in onions, and thus far they have determined the healing
qualities of only a few. These phytonutrients join a host of
other nutrients that contribute to the onion's overall healthful
status. Although all onions are healthful, the general rule for
the more than three hundred varieties is this: the more pungent the onion, the more potent its nutritional value.

- Quercetin, a phytonutrient found in abundance in
  onions, is an antioxidant that helps destroy free radicals, protects and regenerates vitamin E, and helps
  keep LDL levels down.
- A reduction in the risk of colon cancer has also been
  associated with quercitin.
- High blood pressure and high cholesterol may be reduced if you regularly include onions in your diet. Experts say the sulfur compounds, chromium, and vitamin
  B-6 in onions are likely the reason for this benefit.
- Studies show that people who ate the most onions had
  significantly reduced risk for different types of cancer
  compared with people who ate the least onions. The reduced cancer risks were eighty-eight percent for
  esophageal, eighty-four percent for oral cavity and pharyngeal, seventy-three percent for ovarian, seventy-one
  percent for prostate, fifty-six percent for colorectal, and
  twenty-five percent for breast.
- The anti-inflammatory components in onions, especially quercitin and isothiocyanates, benefit people who
  have inflammatory conditions such as arthritis, asthma,
  bronchitis, bursitis, fibromyalgia, and shingles.

How to Select and Store

Choose white, brown, or red onions that are firm, hard, and dry. Pass over any onions that have a soft neck or fresh sprouts. At home, keep onions in a cool, dry, dark place that has good air circulation. Onions should be stored alone; do not put with potatoes, fruits, or vegetables because these other foods, especially potatoes, emit a gas that causes onions to spoil rapidly.

RED ONION SALSA
Makes 3 cups
3 medium red onions, halved, leave skins on
¼ cup olive oil
¼ cup balsamic vinegar
2 Tbs white wine vinegar
1 tsp red pepper flakes
1 cup whole pitted black olives
2 Tbs fresh oregano leaves

Place onion halves cut side down in a shallow pan. Bake at 425 degrees for 30 minutes or until the onions are slightly soft. When they are cool, discard the skins and trim the stems. Place onions in a food processor with the oil, vinegars, and red pepper flakes. Process until coarsely chopped. Add olives and oregano and process 2–4 seconds.

SWEET ONION DRESSING
Makes ¾ cup
3 tbs orange juice
¼ cup minced sweet onion
2 Tbs white wine vinegar
2 tsp prepared brown mustard
2 tsp honey
⅓ cup olive oil

Whisk all ingredients together and chill before using.

ORANGES

When it comes to popular fruit in the United States, oranges come in near the top of the list, but they definitely outdistance their nearest competitors—tomatoes, bananas, and apples—when it comes to vitamin C content. Indeed, some say oranges are the poster child for this vitamin.

Oranges originated several thousand years ago in Southeast Asia and were gradually introduced to other parts of the world by traders. Around the fifteenth century, sweet oranges were brought to Europe, and Christopher Columbus brought seeds to the New World during his second voyage. Those seeds were the beginning of a booming orange industry in the United States, which is dominated by Florida and California. Oranges are also grown in large numbers in Brazil, Mexico, Spain, China, and Israel.

Orange Nutrition
Serving Size: one 2 ⅝-inch diameter
Calories: 62
Protein: 1.3 g
Total Fat: 0.2 g
Carbohydrate: 15.4 g
Fiber: 3 g
Cholesterol: 0 mg
Vitamin C: 69.7 mg, 85% DRI
Folate: 39 mcg, 9% DRI

Health Benefits
Both oranges and orange juice are excellent sources of various phytonutrients, including beta-carotene, flavonoids, and carotenoids, and also provide a fair amount of B vitamins and several minerals. Here's what oranges have to offer.

• Herperidin, a much-researched flavonone in oranges, can lower high blood pressure and cholesterol, and reduce inflammation. Be sure to eat the inner white pulp of the orange, because that's where most of this phytonutrient is found.

- Oranges provide carotenoids, alpha-cryptoxanthin, and zeaxanthin, phytonutrients which protect against development of rheumatoid arthritis, according to the European Prospective Investigation of Cancer Incidence (EPIC)-Norfolk study.
- Nearly fifty studies show that a diet high in citrus provides a forty to fifty percent reduced risk of cancer of the esophagus, stomach, mouth, larynx, and pharynx, according to a 2003 report by the Commonwealth Scientific and Industrial Research Organisation.
- Orange peels contain polymethoxylated flavones (PMFs), which may lower cholesterol more effectively than some prescription drugs, according to a report in the *Journal of Agricultural and Food Chemistry*. The most common PMFs, tangeretin and nobiletin, are found in oranges and tangerines. Adding a tablespoon of grated orange peel (organic) to salads, dressings, yogurt, or other foods daily may help lower your cholesterol.
- Vitamin C prevents free radical damage that triggers inflammation associated with arthritis, asthma, bursitis, fibromyalgia, and heart disease.

How to Select and Store

Shop for oranges that are heavy and firm, with smoothly textured rinds. Avoid fruit that is soft or dry. At home, store oranges in the refrigerator or at room temperature; they should last about two weeks with either case. Keep the oranges loose; placing them in a plastic bag may promote the formation of mold.

ORANGE YAMS
Serves 6
1½ lbs sweet potatoes, cooked, peeled and cut into ¼ inch thick slices

2 oranges, peeled and cut into slices
½ orange, grated peel and juice
2 tsp cornstarch
¼ cup margarine
¼ cup light brown sugar, packed
¼ tsp pumpkin pie spice
¼ cup walnut halves

In an 8-inch square baking pan, arrange the potato slices and orange slices; they will overlap. In a small saucepan, gradually blend the orange juice into the cornstarch; add the margarine, sugar, peel, and pumpkin pie spice. Cover and cook over medium heat, stirring occasionally until thickened. Pour over the potatoes and oranges. Sprinkle with the nuts and bake for 15 minutes at 375° F.

TOPSY TURVY SALAD
Serves 6
2 tomatoes, chopped into ½-inch cubes
1 cup red bell pepper, chopped into ½-inch cubes
1 zucchini, chopped into ½-inch cubes
⅓ cup finely chopped red onion
3 large oranges, peeled and cut into ½-inch cubes

Dressing:

2 Tbs orange juice
1 Tbs lemon juice
1 Tbs balsamic vinegar
1 Tbs olive oil
2 Tbs shredded fresh basil leaves
1 clove garlic, minced
½ tsp each salt and ground black pepper

Place all the fruits and vegetables in a bowl. Combine all the dressing ingredients in a shaker bottle and shake vigorously. Pour dressing over fruits and vegetables and chill for one hour before serving.

PAPAYA

Christopher Columbus called papaya the "fruit of the angels," which may have been a reference to its heavenly, smooth consistency and sweet flavor. Papayas were once considered exotic, but they are now readily available year-round in many areas of the United States. Both the orange flesh, often brightened with yellow or pink hues, and the black seeds are edible, and an outstanding source of vitamin C and phytonutrients.

Papayas are native to Central America and were brought to other subtropical areas including Africa, the Philippines, and India, by early explorers. The fruit was introduced to the United States in the twentieth century, and Hawaii has been a major producer of papayas since the 1920s. Today papayas are grown mainly in the United States, Mexico, and Puerto Rico.

Papaya Nutrition
Serving Size: 1 large: 5¾" long × 3¼" dia.
Calories: 148
Protein: 2.3 g
Total Fat: 0.5 g
Carbohydrates: 37.3 g
Fiber: 6.8 g
Cholesterol: 0 mg
Calcium: 91 mg, 9% DRI
Folate: 144 mcg, 36% DRI
Vitamin A: 4,157 IU, 16% DRI
Vitamin C: 235 g, 287% DRI
Potassium: 977 mg, 28% DRI

Health Benefits
The papaya is an excellent source of antioxidants and various phytonutrients, plus it contains unique protein-digesting enzymes. Consider adding this healthful fruit to your menu on a regular basis.

• The high antioxidant concentrations (vitamins A [beta-carotene] and C) in papayas interfere with the oxidation of cholesterol, which in turn helps prevent atherosclerosis, heart disease, and stroke.

- Vitamins A and C boost the immune system, making it more efficient at preventing infections such as colds, flu, ear aches, gingivitis, and urinary tract infections.
- The fiber in papayas helps lower cholesterol levels and reduce the risk of colon cancer by binding to toxins in the colon and removing them.
- Special enzymes in papaya (papain and chymopapain) reduce inflammation, which makes this fruit useful if you have asthma, arthritis, bursitis, fibromyalgia, or heart disease.
- Papain and chymopapain also aid digestion, and thus provide relief for conditions such as heartburn, irritable bowel syndrome, and ulcers.
- Studies show that vitamins A and C and the carotenoids can help prevent age-related macular degeneration, especially the type associated with vision loss.

How to Select and Store

If you are in the market for papayas that are ready to eat, look for fruit that is slightly soft and that has a reddish-orange skin. Papayas with yellow patches will take a few days to ripen, and green papayas are good for cooking only. Presence of a few black spots on the skin will not affect the taste.

To ripen papayas, leave them at room temperature for a few days. To speed up the process, place them in a paper bag with a banana. Store ripe papayas in the refrigerator and eat them within one or two days for best flavor.

PAPAYA DELIGHT
Serves 4
1 large mango, peeled, seeded, and halved
1 large papaya, peeled, seeded, and halved
1 avocado, peeled, pitted, and diced
3 Tbs balsamic vinegar
1 Tbs margarine

¼ cup blanched slivered almonds
1 tsp brown sugar
1 head romaine lettuce, torn into small pieces

Place half of the mango and half of the papaya into a blender with the vinegar. Puree until smooth and set aside. Melt margarine in a small skillet and brown the almonds. Add brown sugar and stir to coat. Remove from heat and pour the candied almonds onto waxed paper and separate them to avoid clumps. Place romaine lettuce in a large bowl with the diced avocado. Cube the remaining mango and papaya and place in the bowl. Drizzle the pureed fruit over the salad and sprinkle with the candied almonds.

PAPAYA BOATS
Serves 4
1 cup fat-free plain yogurt
¼ cup walnuts, chopped
¼ cup raisins
1 cup chopped fresh strawberries
2 medium papayas, cut in half lengthwise and seeded
2 Tbs honey (optional)

Combine yogurt, walnuts, raisins, and strawberries, and mix gently. Spoon the mixture into the papaya halves and drizzle with honey if desired.

PARSLEY

Parsley, reportedly the world's most popular herb, is native to the Mediterranean area of southern Europe. Ancient people used the greens for medicinal purposes, and the Greeks believed parsley was sacred. "Parsley" is from a Greek word meaning "rock celery," which is appropriate because parsley is a relative of celery.

It wasn't until probably the Middle Ages that parsley was used as a food. The two main types of parsley are curly and

Italian flat leaf. The flat variety is more fragrant and less bitter than the curly type.

Parsley Nutrition

Serving Size: 2 Tbs fresh vs. 2 Tbs. dried
Calories: 2 / 8
Protein: 0.2 g / 0.7 g
Total Fat: 0 g / 0 g
Carbohydrates: 0.5 g / 1.5 g
Fiber: 0.2 g / 1 g
Cholesterol: 0 g / 0 g
Vitamin A: 640 IU, 25% DRI / 326 IU, 13% DRI
Vitamin C: 10 mg, 8.2% DRI / 4 mg, 5% DRI
Vitamin K: 124 mcg, 118% AI / 43 mcg, 41% AI

Health Benefits

Parsley is often ignored—pushed to the side of the plate or tossed away completely—and certainly unappreciated for its health benefits. Besides providing good levels of vitamins A and K, parsley also has several unusual, helpful components: volatile oils (e.g., myristicin, limonene, eugenol, alpha-thujene) and flavonoids (apiin, apigenin, crisoeriol, luteolin). Let's take a closer look.

- Parsley's volatile oils can inhibit tumor formation, especially in the lungs, based on several animal studies.
- The flavonoids in parsley, especially luteolin, help prevent cell damage associated with various diseases, including asthma, atherosclerosis, cancer, diabetes, glaucoma, heart disease, and macular degeneration.
- The combination of vitamin A (beta-carotene) and the flavonoids in parsley boosts the immune system and can help prevent bronchitis, colds, flu, ear infections, and other immune system assaults.
- Vitamin K helps maintain bone density—and thus helps prevent osteoporosis—because it activates osteocalcin, a major protein in bone. Some experts believe vitamin K may help prevent the breakdown of bone.

- Vitamin K may also relieve heavy menstrual flow and/or menstrual pain associated with PMS and/or menopause.

How to Select and Store

Fresh parsley is superior to dried when it comes to flavor and nutritional value. Choose deep green fresh parsley that looks crisp. Whether you choose fresh or dried, buy organic. Store fresh parsley in a plastic bag in the refrigerator. If the parsley begins to wilt, sprinkle it with a small amount of water and return it to the refrigerator.

PARSLEY SOUP

Serves 3–4
1 Tbs peanut or sesame oil
1 large onion, chopped
2 celery stalks, chopped
4 oz fresh parsley, roughly chopped
4 tsp wheat flour
3 cups vegetable broth
Salt and pepper to taste

Heat the oil in a skillet and add the onion, celery, and parsley. Cook until soft, then stir in the flour. Cook for a minute or two before adding the broth. Simmer for 25 minutes, then allow the soup to cool. Puree in a blender. Reheat and season when ready to serve.

PARSLEY PESTO

Makes enough pesto for 5–6 servings of pasta
½ cup chopped walnuts, toasted
¼ cup virgin olive oil
1 cup packed fresh parsley
¼ cup vegetable broth
1 Tbs unseasoned bread crumbs
6 cloves garlic, peeled
½ tsp salt

In a food processor, process all ingredients until smooth. Use with pasta or vegetables.

PEAS

Children in ancient Rome and Greece may have been told to "eat your peas," because this vegetable dates back to those times. The Chinese were likely the first to eat both the seeds and the pods, while other cultures focused on the seeds alone. French King Louis XIV made peas popular in the seventeenth century, and colonists in the New World counted peas among the first vegetables they enjoyed in America. Today's garden peas most likely evolved from the field peas native to Europe and central Asia millennia ago.

Garden peas, snow peas, and sugar snap peas (the latter are a cross between the first two) are the most popular pea varieties. The largest commercial producers of fresh peas today are the United States, Great Britain, China, India, and Hungary.

Pea Nutrition
Serving Size: 1 cup cooked fresh vs. 1 cup canned vs. 1 cup frozen (cooked)
Calories: 134 / 118 / 124
Protein: 8.6 g / 7.5 g / 8.2 g
Total Fat: 0.4 g / 0.6 g / 0.4 g
Carbohydrate: 25 g / 20.5 g / 22.8 g
Fiber: 8.8 g / 7 g / 8.8 g
Cholesterol: 0 mg / 0 mg / 0 mg
Copper: 0.3 mg, 33% DRI / 0.1 mg, 11% DRI / 0.1 mg, 11% DRI
Folate: 101 mcg, 25% DRI / 37 mcg, 9% DRI / 96 mcg, 23% DRI
Iron: 2.5 mg, 18% DRI / 1.6 mg, 12% DRI / 2.5 mg, 18% DRI
Niacin: 3.2 mg, 25% DRI / 1.2 mg 8% DRI / 2.3 mg, 16% DRI
Manganese: 0.8 mg, 40% DRI / 0.5 mg, 25% DRI / 0.5 mg, 25% DRI

Vitamin B-6: 0.3 mg, 20% DRI / 0.1 mg, 7% DRI / 0.2 mg, 13% DRI

Vitamin C: 23 mg, 26% DRI / 16 mg, 20% DRI / 16 mg, 20% DRI

Vitamin K: 41.4 mcg, 39% AI / 36 mcg, 34% AI / 39 mcg, 37% AI

Riboflavin: 0.2 mg, 16% DRI / 0.13 mg, 11% DRI / 0.16 mg, 13% DRI

Thiamin: 0.4 mg, 33% DRI / 0.21 mg, 18% DRI / 0.25, 20% DRI

Zinc: 1.9 mg, 21% DRI / 1.2 mg, 13% DRI / 1.9 mg, 21% DRI

Health Benefits

Peas don't get enough respect: these little green globes are packed with healthy amounts of nutrients that are important for a variety of health concerns.

- Peas are good for bone health: vitamin K activates osteocalcin, a critical bone protein, and helps prevent osteoporosis; folic acid and vitamin B-6 help to reduce high levels of homocysteine, a substance that can hinder the development of bone.
- Green peas can help fight fatigue and boost energy, which is important if you have anemia, fibromyalgia, heart disease, or PMS, or if you are experiencing menopause. That's because green peas provide iron and B vitamins—thiamin, riboflavin, niacin, and vitamin B-6—which are crucial for metabolism.
- Your heart benefits from peas: the high levels of folic acid and vitamin B-6 are important for optimal heart function, while vitamin K helps prevent the formation of clots that can cause heart attack and stroke.

How to Select and Store

Only about five percent of the peas consumed in the United States are fresh; the majority are frozen or canned. If you treat yourself to fresh garden peas, look for firm, velvety smooth, and rounded pods of medium green color. Avoid pods that are yellow or spotted with gray. Fresh peas should be displayed in a refrigerated case because heat speeds up the conversion of their sugar into starch. Snow peas have flat pods, but you should be able to see the shape of the peas through the pod. Choose shiny, small pods because they are usually sweeter. Snap peas should snap when opened and have firm, plump seeds.

Refrigerate fresh peas in a loosely closed bag. Eat them within two to three days to enjoy the freshest flavor.

SNAP PEAS AND SHALLOTS
Serves 4
1 lb sugar snap peas, trimmed
1 large shallot, halved and sliced thin
2 tsp virgin olive oil
¼ tsp salt
Ground black pepper
2 Tbs soy bacon bits

Preheat the oven to 475° F. Toss the peas, shallot, oil, salt, and pepper in a bowl. Place the mixture on a baking sheet and spread to a single layer. Roast in the oven for 12 to 14 minutes, stirring the mixture halfway through the cooking process. Sprinkle with bacon bits and serve.

TANGY SNAP PEAS
Serves 6
1 lb fresh or frozen sugar snap peas
1 small onion, sliced
3 Tbs water
4 tsp sugar
⅛ tsp pepper
1 tsp cornstarch
2 Tbs cider vinegar

In a microwave-safe bowl, combine the peas, onion, and 2 Tbs water. Cover and cook for 5 to 7 minutes, stirring twice. Drain. In a small microwave-safe bowl, combine the sugar, cornstarch, and pepper, stir in the vinegar and remaining water until smooth. Cook, uncovered, for 30–45 seconds or until thickened, stirring once. Add to pea mixture and toss.

PEARS

Pears belong to the rose family, and count apples and quince among their relatives. The origin of pears is unclear: some experts say pears have been around since the Stone Age; others believe they were first cultivated in western Asia about three thousand years ago. Pears were much loved by the French, especially King Louis XIV, and the American colonists imported their pears from France until they got their own trees established.

Of the more than 3,000 known varieties of pears, only a few are cultivated in great numbers around the world. Some of those varieties include bosc, Bartlett, Anjou, comice, and seckel. Most of the world's pear supply is grown in China, Italy, and the United States.

Pear Nutrition
Serving Size: 1 medium
Calories: 103
Protein: 0.7 g
Total Fat: 0.2 g
Carbohydrates: 27.5 g
Fiber: 5.5 g
Cholesterol: 0 mg
Copper: 0.15 mg, 15% DRI

Health Benefits
At first glance, the nutritional information on pears is not overly impressive, but this tasty fruit has some interesting features. Let's look.

- Pears provide copper, a mineral that is a critical part of superoxide dismutase (SOD) and a key player in preventing cell damage. Thus copper may protect against a wide range of health issues, including atherosclerosis, cancer, heart disease, and osteoporosis.

• Copper is important in the prevention and treatment of anemia, because it works with iron to form hemoglobin.

• Pears are less likely to cause adverse reactions, which makes them a possible good choice as the first fruit for infants.

• The abundance of fiber in pears helps prevent constipation, promotes regularity, helps reduce cholesterol levels, and aids the removal of toxins from the intestinal tract, which helps prevent colon cancer, diverticular disease, and irritable bowel syndrome.

How to Select and Store

Pears perish very quickly once they are ripe. Shop for firm pears that have a smooth skin. Pears with brown speckled patches may indicate more flavorful fruit.

To ripen pears, keep them at room temperature. When the skin yields to gentle pressure, the fruit is ripe. Refrigerate any ripe fruit you do not plan to eat immediately. To speed up ripening, place pears in a paper bag, turn them several times a day, and keep them at room temperature. Pears tend to absorb smells, so keep them away from strong-smelling foods.

GRANOLA PEARS
Serves 8
4 Tbs unsalted butter
4 Bartlett pears, halved and cored
2 Tbs lemon juice
1½ cups granola (with almonds and dried cranberries)
⅓ cup maple syrup

Preheat oven to 375 degrees. Butter a 9 × 13" glass baking dish with 1 Tbs butter. Add the pear halves, round side down. Drizzle the pears with lemon juice and fill with granola. Set aside. In a small saucepan, heat the syrup and the remaining butter. Spoon the mixture over the prepared pears. Bake for 40 minutes or until the pears are tender. Baste several times with the juice in the pan.

PEAR SALSA
Serves 4
2 ripe Bartlett pears, diced
2 Tbs dry currants
¼ small red onion, finely diced
½ medium yellow pepper, diced
½ jalapeno pepper, finely diced
1 clove garlic, minced
2 tsp olive oil
Juice from 2 limes
Pinch cayenne pepper
Salt to taste

Combine all ingredients and chill before serving.

PINEAPPLE

Pineapple is a tropical fruit that is believed to have originated in Paraguay. Explorers and traders in South America during the fifteenth and sixteenth centuries carried the fruit back to their native countries, and soon the fruit was being enjoyed as far away as Australia and China. George Washington reportedly grew pineapples in his greenhouse.

Today, about one-third of the world's production of pineapple and sixty percent of the canned fruit comes from Hawaii. Other countries that produce pineapple include Costa Rica, Mexico, Honduras, South Africa, Taiwan, Dominican Republic, Ivory Coast, India, Ecuador, and Australia, among others.

Pineapple Nutrition
Serving Size: 1 cup chunks
Calories: 82
Protein: 0.9 g

Total Fat: 0.2 g
Carbohydrates: 21.6 g
Fiber: 2.3 g
Cholesterol: 0 mg
Copper: 0.18 mg, 21% DRI
Manganese: 1.5 mg, 75% DRI
Vitamin C: 79 mg, 96% DRI

Health Benefits

Pineapple is an unusual-looking fruit that offers several unordinary benefits. For example:

- Pineapple contains a group of enzymes called bromelain, which block the formation of kinins which in turn can help reduce inflammation associated with arthritis, asthma, bursitis, gout, sore throat, and sinusitis. To relieve inflammation, eat pineapple on an empty stomach.
- Bromelain also aids in digestion, and can help prevent or relieve heartburn when it is eaten with or after meals.
- Manganese is an important mineral in the prevention of osteoporosis and chronic fatigue.
- Pineapple stimulates the kidneys, assists in removing toxins from the body, and acts as a diuretic, which can relieve symptoms of PMS, menopause, and urinary tract infections.
- The high vitamin C content in pineapple is a real boost to the immune system in its fight against bacterial and viral infections (e.g., bronchitis, colds, flu, gingivitis, herpes, urinary tract infections) and as an antioxidant to help prevent cell damage.

How to Select and Store

Shop for pineapples that are heavy for their size and with "eyes" that are slightly separated. Avoid pineapples that have soft spots or sunken, dark eyes. Pineapple can be stored at room temperature or in the refrigerator. At room temperature pineapples will get softer but will not ripen. Store any cut pineapple in plastic in the refrigerator, where it should keep for three to four days.

PINEAPPLE SQUASH
Serves 6
1 large acorn squash
2 tsp cinnamon
1 tsp nutmeg
½ tsp allspice
½ tsp ginger
¾ cup chopped pineapple

Cut the squash in half, remove the seeds, and place cut side down on a baking sheet. Bake for 45–60 minutes until soft. (You can also microwave the squash—takes about 7–8 minutes.) Scoop out all the squash and combine it with all the remaining ingredients. Place the mixture back into the halves, place in a casserole dish and bake for 5 minutes until the pineapple bubbles.

GRILLED FRESH PINEAPPLE
Serves 8

Prepare the grill. Cut pineapple lengthwise through the crown but keep the crown attached. Cut each half in half, repeating until you have eight wedges. Grill the wedges on a lightly oiled rack 5 to 6 inches over glowing coals until just charred, about 2 minutes on each cut side.

POMEGRANATES

If you were a world traveler, you might see wild pomegranates growing in Iran and northern India, as well as cultivated varieties throughout the Middle East, southern Europe, and California. The origins of the pomegranate have been traced back about 3,000 years, and some people say that it was a pomegranate, and not an apple, that tempted Eve.

Pomegranates have a rich history in art, medicine, myth, and religion, and they have long been an important part of the Middle Eastern diet. Much of its appeal is due to its unusual presentation: it has a hard, inedible shell that encases a white inedible membrane that surrounds arils—little orbs filled with sweet juice and an edible seed. Eating a pomegranate takes a little effort, but its unique taste and health benefits make it a wise choice.

Pomegranate Nutrition
Serving Size: 1 fruit
Calories: 105
Protein: 1.5 g
Total Fat: 0 g
Carbohydrates: 26.4 g
Fiber: 1 g
Cholesterol: 0 mg
Potassium: 399 mg
Copper: 0.1 mg

Health Benefits
Pomegranates were often ignored until researchers noted the fruit's possible benefits in the fight against prostate cancer. Here is what this neglected fruit may offer beyond its great taste.

- Increasing evidence indicates that pomegranates have a role in the prevention and treatment of prostate cancer. In a 2006 University of California, Los Angeles, study, for example, men with prostate cancer who drank eight ounces of pomegranate juice daily showed a twelve percent decrease in cell proliferation and a seventeen percent increase in cancer cell death.
- A 2007 *International Journal of Impotence Research* study reported that pomegranate juice may help fight erectile dysfunction. The study was done in men who had mild to moderate erectile dysfunction, and fifty-nine percent reported improvement after drinking the juice during the eight-week treatment.

- Pomegranate juice is an excellent source of three types of polyphenols—tannins, anthocyanins, and ellagic acid—all of which are potent antioxidants. These substances have been associated with the prevention of heart disease and cancer.
- Pomegranates also appear to have anticancer activity against breast cancer cells. A Florida Atlantic University study found that pomegranate extracts inhibited the growth of human breast cancer cells.
- Pomegranate juice is heart-healthy: a 2005 Preventive Medicine Research Institute study showed that eight ounces of pomegranate juice consumed daily for three months improved the amount of oxygen that reached the heart muscles of patients who had coronary heart disease.

How to Select and Store

Shop for fruit that is heavy for its size and has a bright, unblemished skin. Pomegranates will stay fresh in the refrigerator for up to two months, or in a cool, dark place for up to one month.

POMEGRANATE AND CUCUMBER SALAD
Serves 4
½ cup chopped scallions
½ cup chopped fresh mint
1 tsp salt
½ tsp ground pepper
1 cucumber, peeled and diced
Seeds of 2 pomegranates
1 fresh lime, peeled and sliced with inner skin removed

Combine all ingredients in a bowl, toss, and chill before serving.

SPICY POMEGRANATE RELISH
Makes 1½ cups
Seeds from 2 pomegranates, about 1½ cups
½ cup finely chopped red onion
1½ Tbs finely chopped jalapeno pepper

1 Tbs lemon juice
1 Tbs sugar
¼ tsp salt

Toss all ingredients together and chill before using.

PRUNES

To be politically—and gastronomically—correct, the official
name for plums that have been dried has been changed from
prunes to *dried plums*. Hopefully, tossing out the old name will
also help eliminate the somewhat negative image that has been
associated with prunes for many years. Dried plums are naturally sweet and delicious, nutritious, and convenient to eat.

Plums were most likely first dried thousands of years ago in
the area around the Caspian Sea, where European plums originated. In California, the world's leading producer of dried
plums, prune production began in the mid-nineteenth century
when Louis Pellier brought grafts from the Agen variety to the
United States. Today, the Agen plum is one of the best suited
for making dried plums.

Prune Nutrition
Serving Size: ½ cup dried
Calories: 209
Protein: 1.7 g
Total Fat: 0.3 g
Carbohydrates: 56 g
Fiber: 6.2 g
Cholesterol: 0 mg
Copper: 0.49 mg, 53% DRI
Iron: 0.8 mg, 6% DRI
Potassium: 637 mg, 13% DRI

Health Benefits
Dried plums are the source of unique phytonutrients called
neochlorogenic and chlorogenic acid. These substances are a

type of phenol that functions as an antioxidant, but not just any antioxidant. Let's take a closer look at the advantages of eating dried plums.

- Neochlorogenic and chlorogenic acids attack an especially damaging free radical called superoxide anion radical and can also help prevent damage to fats. This latter benefit is very important because cell membranes—including brain cells—are composed largely of fats.
- Dried plums are a good source of potassium, and complement that mineral with a very low amount of sodium, a combination that can be helpful in preventing high blood pressure and protecting against atherosclerosis, stroke, and other cardiovascular conditions.
- The propionic acid produced by the insoluble fiber in dried plums may be partly responsible for the fruit's ability to lower cholesterol levels. Propionic acid inhibits an enzyme that aids in the production of cholesterol. When the enzyme's activity is hindered, cholesterol production declines.
- High fiber can help prevent intestinal conditions such as constipation, diarrhea, diverticular diseases, and irritable bowel syndrome, as well as reduce the risk of colon cancer and hemorrhoids.
- High fiber may help prevent heart disease. A large (nearly 10,000 adults), nineteen-year study found that people who ate the most fiber (21 g daily) had 11 percent less cardiovascular disease and 12 percent less coronary heart disease compared with people who ate the least (5 g daily) fiber.
- Dried plums may increase the absorption of iron into the body, which may help prevent and treat anemia and fatigue.

How to Select and Store

Dried plums are sold already pitted or with their pits. In either case, look for fruit that is plump, soft, and shiny, and that has not been processed with food preservatives such as sulfites.

Keep dried plums in an airtight container as they can dry out or become moldy when they are exposed to air. Store the container in a dark, cool, dry place. Refrigerated dried plums can last up to six months; those in a cupboard should last two to four months.

PRUNE PUREE
Makes 1 cup
1⅓ cups pitted prunes
6 Tbs water

Place prunes and water in a food processor and pulse until the prunes are finely chopped. This mixture can be used in a variety of ways, including the Plum Smoothie recipe below. The puree can also be used as a substitute for fat in many recipes; for example, in place of butter, oil, or margarine in cake, muffin, and quick bread recipes. For recipes that call for butter or margarine, you can replace all or part of the fat with half as much puree. If the recipe calls for oil, replace all or part of the oil with three-fourths as much puree.

PLUM SMOOTHIE
Serves 1
¼ cup plain or vanilla low-fat yogurt
½ cup prune puree
1 medium banana
3 ice cubes

Combine the yogurt, puree, and banana, and process in a food processor or blender. When smooth, add the ice and process to desired consistency.

PUMPKIN SEEDS

Pumpkins have long been a favorite of people in many cultures, yet the seeds themselves are especially celebrated in Mexican cuisine. Native American Indians used both the pumpkin and its seeds as food and medicine, and the colonists took these new foods back to Europe and shared their find on that continent.

The leading producers of pumpkins today are the United States, Mexico, China, and India.

Pumpkin Seed Nutrition

Serving Size: 1 ounce kernels, dried
Calories: 151
Protein: 7 g
Total Fat: 13 g
Carbohydrates: 5 g
Fiber: 1 g
Cholesterol: 0 mg
Iron: 4.2 mg, 32% DRI
Magnesium: 152 mg, 40% DRI
Copper: 0.4 mg, 44% DRI
Zinc: 2.1 mg, 23% DRI

Health Benefits

Here's a look at some of the advantages associated with these nutritious seeds.

- Components found in pumpkin seed oil seem to interrupt the mechanism that triggers the duplication of prostate cells by testosterone and dihydrotestosterone, the factors that cause benign prostatic hypertrophy or BPH. The question is, which components offer this benefit? Pumpkin seeds contain carotenoids, omega-3 fatty acids, and zinc, all of which may be responsible for this benefit.
- The zinc in pumpkin seeds may help improve bone density. In a study published in the *American Journal*

of Clinical Nutrition, experts found a clear relationship between low intake of zinc, low blood levels of zinc, and osteoporosis in nearly four hundred men.

• Pumpkin seeds have a high level of phytosterols (265 mg/3.5 oz of seeds), plant compounds that may reduce cholesterol, boost the immune system, and decrease the risk of some cancers.

• Pumpkin seeds have excellent levels of magnesium, which can be helpful for allergies, chronic fatigue syndrome, fibromyalgia, glaucoma, headache, hemorrhoids, high blood pressure, osteoporosis, Parkinson's disease, and PMS.

• The manganese provided by pumpkin seeds may help if you have osteoporosis, as low levels are found in people who have this disease. Low magnesium levels have also been associated with ear infections.

• The high iron content in pumpkin seeds may help if you have anemia or chronic fatigue syndrome.

How to Select and Store

Pumpkin seeds are generally available in prepackaged containers and in bulk. In either form, be sure the seeds look fresh and have no evidence of damage or mold. If possible, smell the seeds to see if they have a musty or rancid odor. Store pumpkin seeds in an airtight container in the refrigerator. Pumpkin seeds retain their freshness for up to two months, after which time they are still edible but less tasty or crunchy.

HOW TO USE PUMPKIN SEED KERNELS
• Sprinkle on cooked vegetables
• Add to salads
• Stir into hot cereals and rice
• Enjoy as a snack
• Blend into smoothies

MAKE PUMPKIN SEEDS
Seeds extracted from a pumpkin
Water

Salt
Olive oil

Preheat oven to 400° F. Remove the seeds from a pumpkin and rinse them to remove any strings. In a small saucepan add the seeds to water, about 2 cups of water for every half cup of seeds, along with 1 tablespoon of salt for every cup of water. Bring to a boil, let simmer for 10 minutes, then remove from heat and drain. Spread about 1 tablespoon of olive oil on the bottom of a roasting pan. Spread the seeds out in a single layer and bake on the top rack of the oven for 20 minutes or until the seeds begin to brown. Enjoy with the shells on or remove the inner kernels.

QUINOA

Quinoa, although it looks like a grain, is actually a relative of leafy green vegetables like spinach and Swiss chard. The plant has been cultivated in the mountainous regions of Peru, Chile, and Bolivia for more than five millennia and was considered to be sacred by the Incas. Today it is still a major food in the diet of the native Indians, and has gained some popularity among Americans and other people because of its high nutritional content.

Quinoa Nutrition
Serving Size: ¼ cup uncooked
Calories: 159
Protein: 5.6 g
Total Fat: 2.5 g
Carbohydrates: 29.3 g
Fiber: 2.5 g
Cholesterol: 0 mg
Iron: 3.9 mg, 30% DRI
Magnesium: 89 mg, 23% DRI
Manganese: 0.96 mg, 48% DRI
Riboflavin: 0.17 mg, 14% DRI

Health Benefits

One special feature of quinoa is that it is a complete protein, which means it contains all nine essential amino acids. (Most plant protein foods do not meet this goal.) It is also a good source of magnesium, copper, iron, and phosphorus. These and other nutrients make quinoa a healthful food choice.

- Migraine sufferers may benefit from quinoa because of its high magnesium content. Magnesium relaxes blood vessels, and increased intake of this mineral has reduced incidence of migraines.
- Riboflavin assists energy production and has been shown to help reduce the frequency of migraine attacks.
- Magnesium may offer help with high blood pressure, ischemic heart disease, and heart arrhythmias.
- Whole grains like quinoa can help reduce the risk of high blood pressure and heart attack. Researchers followed 21,376 participants for nearly 20 years and found that a daily bowl of whole-grain cereal was associated with a 29 percent reduced risk of heart attack and a 29 percent reduced risk of heart failure.

How to Select and Store

Quinoa is usually available in prepackaged containers and in bulk bins. Regardless of which type you buy, make sure the grain is moisture-free. Store quinoa in an airtight container, either in a cool, dark area or in the refrigerator. Refrigerated quinoa will stay fresh approximately three to six months, slightly less time if kept at room temperature.

QUINOA BREAKFAST

Serves 1–2
½ cup water
¼ cup quinoa
¼ cup steel-cut oats
¼ cup crushed pineapple
1 Tbs blackstrap molasses
Raisins or currants if desired

Rinse the quinoa. Boil and then simmer the quinoa in water and molasses for 10 minutes. Add the oats and fruit (if desired) and simmer for an additional 15 minutes.

QUINOA SOUP
Serves 2
1 14-oz can vegetable broth
½ cup quinoa, rinsed and drained
¼ tsp cayenne pepper
2 cloves garlic, minced
1 cup frozen or fresh corn kernels
1½ Tbs chopped cilantro
1 Tbs lime juice

Place the broth, quinoa, water, cayenne, and garlic in a soup pot and bring to a boil. Reduce heat to medium and cook 10 minutes. Add corn kernels and cook 3 minutes. Add cilantro and cook for 1 minute. Remove from heat and stir in the lime juice. Serve hot or cold.

RADISHES

The radish is a root vegetable that is a member of the mustard family. It is also a cruciferous vegetable, so it counts the cancer-fighting broccoli, cauliflower, kale, and similar vegetables among its relatives.

Although the small, red globe radishes are the most popular and common in the United States, there are four other varieties also seen in the states: black, white icicle, California mammoth white, and daikon (an Asian variety). The daikon is the second most popular radish in the United States, and it is slightly more pungent and juicier than the red variety, but milder than the black.

Radish Nutrition

Red Radishes
Serving Size: 1 cup sliced, raw
Calories: 19

Protein: 1 g
Total Fat: 0 g
Carbohydrates: 4 g
Fiber: 2 g
Cholesterol: 0 mg
Vitamin C: 17 mg, 20% DRI

Daikon

Serving Size: one 7-inch, raw
Calories: 61
Protein: 2 g
Total Fat: 0 g
Carbohydrates: 14 g
Fiber: 5 g
Cholesterol: 0 mg
Vitamin C: 74 mg, 91% DRI
Folate: 95 mcg, 23% DRI
Iron: 1.35 mg, 10% DRI
Potassium: 767 mg, 16% DRI

Health Benefits

Red radishes are a very good source of vitamin C and iodine. Daikons have even more vitamin C than their red relatives, as well as good levels of potassium, folate, and iron.
When it comes to radishes, go beyond red.

- Radishes contain phytonutrients called indoles, which
  may help fight cancers driven by hormones; that is,
  breast, prostate, cervical, and endometrial.
- The high vitamin C and folate content in daikon may
  help strengthen the immune system against infections
  (e.g., bronchitis, colds, ear infections, flu, gingivitis,
  urinary tract infections, vaginitis) and act as a potent
  antioxidant against conditions such as atherosclerosis,
  chronic fatigue syndrome, glaucoma, herpes, psoriasis, and shingles.
- Daikons offer a high level of fiber, which can be helpful in cases of high cholesterol, high blood pressure,

diarrhea, constipation, irritable bowel syndrome, hemorrhoids, and varicose veins.

How to Select and Store

When shopping for red radishes, look for bright, unblemished, firm globes that have short, lively green tops. Before refrigerating them, break off the leaves and put the roots into a plastic bag. They should stay fresh for about one week. Before serving the radishes, soak them in ice water for an hour to make them crisp. If you choose daikons, look for firm roots that are heavy for their size. Remove the tops, refrigerate the roots in a plastic bag, and use within one week.

RADICAL RADISH SOUP
Serves 4–5
5 cups vegetable broth
¼ cup rice vinegar
2 Tbs sugar
¼ tsp cayenne pepper
¼ tsp ground ginger
1 lb cooked turkey, cubed
6 oz sliced radishes (1½ cups)
1½ cups spinach leaves, shredded
⅔ cups thinly sliced green onions

In a large saucepan over medium heat, bring the broth to a boil. Stir in the vinegar, sugar, cayenne, and ginger. Add the remaining ingredients, cover, and let stand 2–3 minutes before serving.

PICKLED DAIKON
Serves 6
½ lb daikon, shredded
1 carrot, shredded
1 Tbs canning salt
1 cup water
¼ cup distilled white vinegar
1 Tbs sugar
1 tsp red pepper flakes (optional)

Put daikon and carrot into a bowl, sprinkle with salt, and mix well. Let stand for 30 minutes. Drain off water and squeeze vegetables as dry as possible. In a small bowl combine vinegar, sugar, and pepper flakes. Place the vegetables in a clean quart jar, add the vinegar mixture, and refrigerate overnight or at least 6–8 hours.

RAISINS

People have dried grapes into raisins since ancient times, and raisins are mentioned in the Old Testament. These dried fruits were so revered by ancient Romans that they used them as currency and as prizes for sporting events.

Today, raisins are popular around the world. The largest commercial producer of raisins is the San Joaquin Valley in California, which has cultivated them since the nineteenth century. The story goes that when a heat wave destroyed the grape harvest in 1873, an enterprising grape grower took the dried grapes to a grocer in San Francisco, who sold them as a special delicacy. The raisins caught on, and since then they have been popular in the United States. Other raisin producers include Australia, Chile, Greece, Iran, and Turkey.

Raisin Nutrition
Serving Size: 1 oz seedless
Calories: 85
Protein: 1 g
Total Fat: 0 g
Carbohydrates: 22 g
Fiber: 1 g
Cholesterol: 0 mg
Copper: 0.09 mg, 10% DRI

Health Benefits
On first glance, raisins don't look overly impressive on the health front because they don't have high levels of any major

nutrients. Yet they are a naturally sweet, high-energy food that is convenient and easy to take anywhere: while hiking, camping, flying, in the car, at work, school, or play. They are also a nutritious food that picky eaters enjoy. Here are a few more advantages:

- Raisins are one of the few foods that provide a good amount of boron, a trace mineral that is important in bone health and osteoporosis. Boron is especially important in postmenopausal women because it reproduces many of the good effects of estrogen, including its ability to help maintain bone density.
- The phytonutrients in raisins, especially oleanolic acid, are very effective in killing bacteria that cause cavities (*Streptococcus mutans*) and gingivitis (*Porphyromonas gingivalis*).

How to Select and Store

If possible, choose raisins in containers that allow you to evaluate their quality to make sure they are moist and undamaged. If the raisins are in another type of container, make sure it is tightly sealed. At home, store raisins in an airtight container in the refrigerator to extend their freshness. They are best when eaten within six months of purchase.

RAISIN CRANBERRY RELISH

Makes about 3 cups
2¼ cups golden raisins
2 cups orange juice
1 cup water
¼ cup lemon juice
⅔ cup sugar
3 cups cranberries, fresh or frozen
1 Tbs finely grated orange peel

In a large saucepan, combine raisins, orange juice, water, lemon juice, and sugar. Bring to a boil, stirring to dissolve the sugar. Reduce heat and simmer for 10 minutes. Add cranberries and orange peel. Return to boil, simmer for 10 minutes. Cool and store in the refrigerator in a covered container, where it will keep for up to 1 month.

RAISIN TAPENADE
Makes 16 appetizers
1 cup raisins
½ cup pitted kalamata olives
1 Tbs virgin olive oil
3 Tbs orange juice
2 Tbs orange zest
16 baguette slices
½ cup low-fat soft goat cheese

In a food processor, pulse raisins, olives, olive oil, orange juice, and zest until it forms a coarse paste. Spread about ½ tablespoon of soft goat cheese on each baguette slice and top with the raisin mixture.

RASPBERRIES

The raspberry is a delicately structured, sweet yet slightly tart berry that dates back to prehistoric times. The most common type is red-pink in color, but they also come in orange, yellow, white, black, and purple. Wild raspberries are believed to have originated in eastern Asia, but there are many varieties native to the Western Hemisphere.

Raspberries were likely first cultivated around 1548 in Europe, and they began to be more widely grown in both Europe and North America in the nineteenth century. Today the major commercial producers of raspberries include Russia, Poland, Yugoslavia, Germany, Chile, and the United States, specifically California.

Raspberry Nutrition
Serving Size: 1 cup, raw
Calories: 64
Protein: 1.5 g
Total Fat: 0.8 g
Carbohydrates: 14.7 g
Fiber: 8 g
Cholesterol: 0 mg
Manganese: 0.8 mg, 40% DRI
Vitamin C: 32 mg, 31% DRI

Health Benefits
Raspberries are rich in various phytonutrients. In fact, raspberries have nearly fifty percent higher antioxidant activity than strawberries, three times that of kiwis, and ten times that of tomatoes. Here are a few of the advantages of including raspberries to your diet.

- Raspberries contain anthocyanins, which have both antioxidant and antimicrobial properties. One advantage of anthocyanins is their ability to prevent growth of *Candida albicans*, a cause of vaginal infections and a contributing cause in irritable bowel syndrome.
- Raspberries may have cancer-prevention qualities. This feature is credited to phytonutrients called ellagitannins, which are almost exclusive to raspberries.
- The high antioxidant power of raspberries makes them strongly recommended for preventing macular degeneration. A study (*Archives of Ophthalmology*) of more than 110,000 adults found that the antioxidant power of fruits is much more effective than that of vegetables in preventing age-related and neovascular macular degeneration.
- The very high fiber content in raspberries may help prevent intestinal conditions, including constipation, diarrhea, hemorrhoids, irregularity, and irritable bowel syndrome.

How to Select and Store

Because raspberries are highly perishable, you should consume them within one to two days of purchase. Look for
berries that you can see clearly in their packaging or buy them
loose. Choose plump, firm, deeply colored berries. Before you
store them in the refrigerator, remove any spoiled fruits. Place
unwashed berries in a container or spread them out on a
paper-towel-lined plate and cover with plastic wrap. They
should remain fresh for up to two days. Do not leave raspberries at room temperature or exposed to sunlight, as they will
spoil more rapidly.

Raspberries freeze very well. To prepare for freezing, wash
the berries very gently, pat dry with a paper towel, arrange
them in a single layer on a flat pan, and place them in the
freezer. Once frozen, place the berries in a heavy plastic bag
and return them to the freezer. They will stay fresh for up to
one year.

RASPBERRY SMOOTHIE
Makes 3 cups
1 cup raspberry juice
1 cup fresh raspberries
½ cup sliced banana, frozen
1 cup plain soy yogurt, frozen
½ cup chopped ice cubes
Place all ingredients into a blender and pulse until smooth.

RASPBERRY SAUCE
Makes about 1 cup
½ cup fresh raspberries
8 oz silken tofu
3 Tbs white wine vinegar
3 Tbs sugar

Place all ingredients into a blender and pulse until smooth.
Use on salads, as a dip, or with poultry.

RED WINE

It's not the alcohol but the antioxidants that provide the real kick—the health kick, that is–when it comes to red wine. Unlike white wine, which is fermented from the pressed juice of grapes alone, red wine is fermented with the seeds, twigs, skins, and leaves of the grape vines, which means the finished product contains much greater quantities of the beneficial phytonutrients found in these plant parts.

Red Wine Nutrition
Serving Size: 5 oz. Cabernet Sauvignon
Calories: 122
Protein: 0 g
Total Fat: 0 g
Carbohydrates: 3.8 g
Fiber: 0 g
Cholesterol: 0 mg

Note: Comparable values for these nutrients are found for other red wines as well, including red table, Burgundy, Zinfandel.

Health Benefits
The health benefits of red wine are related to its high antioxidant content—the polyphenols, anthrocyanidins, and resveratrol, among others. Resveratrol, for example, is about twenty to fifty times as effective as vitamin C alone. Thus red wine presents some interesting nutritional advantages.

- Saponins in red wine may lower cholesterol levels, according to a 2003 University of California Davis study.
- Red wine may help fight cavities, upper respiratory tract infections, and gingivitis, according to a 2007 study published in the *Journal of Agricultural and Food Chemistry*.
- A year-long study of more than 4,000 volunteers found that those who drank more than two glasses of red wine

daily had 44 percent fewer colds than people who did not drink wine. This benefit also did not occur for people who drank beer or spirits.

• Men who drink an average of four to seven glasses of red wine per week are only fifty-two percent as likely to be diagnosed with prostate cancer as those who do not drink red wine. Another study (*International Journal of Cancer*) found that drinking four or more glasses of red wine weekly reduced the risk of prostate cancer by fifty percent, and that wine had the greatest impact on the most aggressive tumors, with a sixty percent reduction in those cases.

• Antioxidants called flavonoids reduce the risk of coronary heart disease by (1) reducing production of low-density ("bad") lipoprotein cholesterol; (2) raising high-density ("good") lipoprotein cholesterol levels; and (3) reducing blood clotting.

• There is evidence that resveratrol may help prevent neurodegenerative diseases such as Parkinson's disease and dementia, according to a 2007 study published in *Mutation Research*.

• A University of Missouri-Columbia study has found that red wine has antimicrobial properties that fight various disease-causing agents, including *Helicobacter pylori*, which causes ulcers.

How to Select and Store

When choosing a red wine for its flavonoid content, your best bets are Cabernet Sauvignon, Petit Syrah, and Pinot Noir, according to a study at the University of California, Davis. Both Merlots and red zinfandels have lower levels of flavonoids than the aforementioned wines. Generally, the drier the wine, the higher the level of flavonoids. White wine has significantly smaller amounts of flavonoids.

Store wine in a cool place and out of direct sunlight. If you do not plan to use the wine within a few weeks, store the bottle on its side so you keep the cork moist and thus the bottle airtight.

PEARS IN RED WINE
Serves 4
4 medium pears
⅓ cup sugar
1 Tbs black peppercorns
5 whole cloves
1 3-inch cinnamon stick
1 750-milliliter bottle dry red wine
¼ cup crumbled blue cheese (optional)

Peel and core the pears, cut each pear in half lengthwise and set aside. In a skillet, place the peppercorns, cloves, cinnamon, and wine, and bring to a boil over medium heat. Arrange the pears, cut sides down, in a single layer in the skillet. Cover, reduce heat, and simmer for 10 minutes. Turn pears over and simmer for an additional 10 minutes. Remove the pears and place in a shallow dish. Bring the wine mixture to a boil and cook for 20 minutes or until reduced to ¾ cup. Strain the mixture through a sieve and discard the spices. Pour the wine over the pears and chill for 8 hours. Serve with crumbled cheese if desired.

RED WINE SPRITZERS
Serves 4–6
½ pint blackberries
½ pint raspberries
1 bottle 750 ml, dry red table wine
1 quart sparkling water or seltzer, chilled

Fill the bottom of large wine glasses with a mixture of the berries. Pour wine in to cover and let stand 10 minutes. Top glasses with seltzer when you are ready to serve.

SEA VEGETABLES

Sea vegetables (also referred to as seaweed) have been a staple food among the Japanese and Chinese for millennia. In fact, most cultures that are located near salt water have included sea vegetables in their diet since ancient times, including Scotland, Ireland, New Zealand, the Pacific Islands, and coastal South American countries. The high nutritional value of sea vegetables have brought them to the attention of Western cultures, where they are slowly being accepted.

"Sea vegetables" is actually a slight misnomer, as some of these algae (sea vegetables are neither plants nor animals) grow in fresh water. Among the more common sea vegetables are agar, arame, hijiki, kelp, nori, spirulina, and wakame. Today Japan is the largest producer and exporter of sea vegetables.

Sea Vegetable Nutrition

Agar (dried)
Serving Size: 1 oz.
Calories: 86
Protein: 1.7 g
Total Fat: 0 g
Carbohydrates: 23 g
Fiber: 2.2 g
Cholesterol: 0 mg
Copper: 0.17 mg, 19% DRI
Folate: 162 mcg, 40% DRI
Iron: 6 mg, 46% DRI
Magnesium: 216 mg, 56% DRI
Zinc: 1.6 mg, 17% DRI

Wakame
Serving Size: 3.5 oz., raw
Calories: 45
Protein: 3 g
Total Fat: 0.6 g
Carbohydrates: 9 g
Fiber: 0.5 g
Cholesterol: 0 mg
Calcium: 150 mg, 12% DRI

Copper: 0.3 mg, 33% DRI
Folate: 196 mg, 49% DRI
Iron: 2.18 mg, 16% DRI
Manganese: 1.4 mg, 70% DRI

Health Benefits

The wide range of minerals in sea vegetables is the same as the ones found in human blood. Sea vegetables are also a good source of various plant compounds. Let's explore the benefits of all these elements.

- Phytonutrients called lignans can inhibit the process by which cancer can spread and grow. Lignans can also inhibit the synthesis of estrogen in fat cells, which is a key factor in the risk for breast cancer.
- Folate has been associated with a significantly reduced risk for colon cancer, and some sea vegetables (e.g., wakame, dried agar) have a high amount of this B vitamin.
- Nature's richest source of iodine is sea vegetables, and this nutrient is essential for the manufacture of the thyroid hormones thyroxine and triiodothyronine. Because these hormones regulate metabolism in every cell of the body, an iodine deficiency can have a dramatic negative impact on your health.
- Most sea vegetables contain a fair amount of iron, which can be helpful for preventing and treating anemia and fatigue.
- Some sea vegetables contain unique substances called fucans, which can reduce the body's inflammatory response. That means these algaes may help relieve symptoms of arthritis, asthma, bursitis, fibromyalgia, and heart disease.
- For women who have symptoms of menopause, the magnesium in sea vegetables can help restore sleep, while the lignans, which can act as very weak estrogen, may relieve hot flashes and other menopausal symptoms.

How to Select and Store

Sea vegetables are available as flakes, powder, and sheets, but regardless of the form you buy, they should be in tightly sealed packages to avoid moisture. Store sea vegetables in tightly sealed containers once you open them, and keep them at room temperature, which should keep them fresh for several months.

SEAFOOD SOUP
Serves 4
1 piece of kelp, 4"×4"
3 oz soba noodles (or your favorites)
6 cups water
½ cup carrot strips, julienned
¼ lb extra firm tofu, diced
¼ cup red pepper strips
3 Tbs light miso
1 tsp grated ginger

Simmer the kelp in the water for 8–10 minutes. Remove the kelp and reserve the broth. Slice into thin 2- to 3-inch-long strips and put the strips into the broth. Add the carrots and noodles and simmer on low for 2–3 minutes until the noodles are slightly underdone. Puree miso in a cup with some of the broth. Add the tofu, red pepper strips, ginger, and miso to the pot and stir. Simmer for 2–3 minutes and serve. Garnish with scallions if desired.

WALDORF-DULSE SALAD
Serves 6
1 head red leaf lettuce, chopped
1 cup chopped dulse
2 apples cut into chunks
3 grated carrots
1 cup chopped celery
½ cup chopped walnuts
Dressing: ⅔ cup olive oil
Juice of 1 lemon
4 Tbs soy sauce

Combine all the salad ingredients. In a shaker bottle, combine the dressing ingredients, shake well, and pour over salad. Let the salad marinate for 20 minutes to allow the dulse to absorb moisture and soften.

SALMON

Salmon are a popular fish for their taste and their nutritional value. People have likely been eating salmon ever since they discovered the fish in their waterways. At one point during their lifetime these fascinating fish travel thousands of miles to return to their birthplace, where they spawn and then die.

The specific life cycles and nutritional values of salmon differ among species, and flesh color also varies, from pink to orange and red. Most of the salmon in today's market comes from Alaska, eastern Canada, the Pacific Northwest, Norway, and Greenland.

Salmon Nutrition

Atlantic salmon: farmed vs wild
   Serving Size: 3 oz cooked
   Calories: 175 / 155
   Protein: 19 g / 21.6 g
   Total Fat: 10.5 g / 6.9 g
   Carbohydrates: 0 g / 0 g
   Fiber: 0 g / 0 g
   Cholesterol: 54 mg / 60 mg
   Niacin: 6.8 mg, 45% DRI / 8.6 mg, 57% DRI
   Selenium: 35 mg, 63% DRI / 40 mg, 73% DRI
   Vitamin B-12: 2.4 mcg, 100% DRI / 2.6 mcg, 108% DRI

Coho: farmed vs wild
   Serving Size: 3 oz cooked
   Calories: 151 / 156
   Protein: 26 g / 23 g
   Total Fat: 7 g / 6.3 g

Carbohydrates: 0 g / 0 g
Fiber: 0 g / 0 g
Cholesterol: 54 mg / 48 mg
Niacin: 6.3 mg, 42% DRI / 6.6 mg, 44% DRI
Selenium: 12 mg, 22% DRI / 39 mg, 71% DRI
Vitamin B-12: 2.7 mcg, 113% DRI / 3.8 mcg, 158% DRI

Health Benefits

Experts generally agree that salmon is a healthy food choice, especially because of its high omega-3 fatty acid content. The controversy is over whether wild-caught or farmed salmon is the healthier and/or safer choice. Many studies, including one conducted by researchers at Indiana University in 2004, have found higher levels of toxins, including carcinogenic chemicals called polychlorinated biphenyls (PCBs; up to sixteen times greater), in farmed than in wild salmon. Farmed salmon also have higher amounts of saturated fat and lower levels of beneficial omega-3 fatty acids, although not all studies agree with the findings regarding omega-3 levels. Farmed or wild, salmon is still a very good source of omega-3 fatty acids.

- Salmon promotes heart health because omega-3 fatty acids prevent platelets from forming clots; niacin helps lower elevated cholesterol; and vitamin B-12 helps reduce homocysteine, an amino acid that damages blood vessels.
- Omega-3 fatty acids help reduce blood pressure, and thus reduce the risk of heart attack and stroke.
- Eating salmon at least twice a week may significantly reduce the progression of atherosclerosis in post-menopausal women who have diabetes, according to a 2004 study published in the *American Journal of Clinical Nutrition*.
- Swedish researchers have found that men who eat salmon once or twice per week are at least forty-three percent less likely to develop prostate cancer than men who do not eat salmon.
- In a study of more than ten thousand cancer patients,

researchers found that eating more fish correlated with a reduced risk of cancer of the pancreas, mouth, esophagus, stomach, colon, and rectum.

- Fish consumption and the resulting increase in omega-3 fatty acid levels in the blood is associated with significantly less memory loss and mental decline over time.
- A diet high in omega-3 fatty acids provides significant protection against early and late age-related macular degeneration (ARMD). One study found a forty-two percent reduced risk of early ARMD among people who ate omega-3 rich fish at least once per week compared with those who ate little or no fish. Those who ate fish at least three times per week saw a seventy-five percent reduction.
- Several studies show a connection between increased rates of depression and decreased consumption of omega-3 fatty acids.
- A large Dutch study found that a high intake of fish was associated with a sixty-six percent reduction in the risk of being asthmatic.

How to Select and Store

Salmon is sold fresh as a whole fish, fillet, or steak, or it is available frozen, canned, dried, or smoked. Whether you choose wild or farmed salmon (see above), only buy fish that is in a refrigerated (or frozen) case and is being sold by a reputable dealer or store. Transport the fish home in a cooler. Once at home, rinse and rewrap the fish, place it on paper towels, then put it in a plastic bag or tightly covered container. Place in the coldest part of the refrigerator or in the freezer. Use refrigerated fish within two to three days. Frozen fish can keep for several months.

LEMON GARLIC SALMON
Serves 2
2 six-oz salmon fillets
2 Tbs margarine
2 tsp minced garlic

 1 tsp lemon pepper
Lemon juice

Melt the margarine in a skillet and sauté the garlic. Season the salmon on both sides with lemon pepper. Place the fillets in the pan and cook until it flakes when tested with a fork. Turn fillets midway through cooking to brown on both sides. Sprinkle with lemon juice.

SALMON DIP
8 oz canned salmon
2 Tbs toasted sesame seeds
2 Tbs green onions, minced
½ cup plain low-fat yogurt
½ tsp ground ginger

Drain and flake the salmon. Combine all the ingredients in a bowl and mix well. Cover the bowl and chill for 2 hours before serving.

SOYBEANS/TOFU

The slightly nutty tasting soybean is the most widely grown legume in the world. It is highly regarded for its significant protein and nutrient content, and is also one of the most researched, healthful foods available today.

Experts believe soybeans were first domesticated around the eleventh century BC, in northern China, and then gradually made their way throughout China and Korea. By the sixteenth century, soybeans had made their way throughout Asia and much of India and were accepted as a staple in the diet. Europeans who visited China and Japan during the late sixteenth and early seventeenth centuries were intrigued by soybeans and the foods made from them, namely tofu, miso, and soy sauce, and brought samples back with them. Soybeans reached the United States around 1765, when a former seaman and Georgia farmer, Samuel Bowen, brought soybeans from China and planted them on his plantation. Today the major soybean producing nations are the United States, Brazil, Argentina, and China.

Soybean Nutrition

Soybeans
Serving Size: 1 cup cooked
Calories: 298
Protein: 28.6 g
Total Fat: 15.4 g
Carbohydrates: 17 g
Fiber: 10.3 g
Cholesterol: 0 mg
Calcium: 175 mg, 18% DRI
Folate: 93 mcg, 23% DRI
Iron: 8.8 mg, 59% DRI
Magnesium: 148 mg, 39% DRI
Riboflavin: 0.5 mg, 42% DRI
Thiamin: 0.27 mg, 23% DRI
Vitamin B-6: 0.4 mg, 27% DRI

Tofu, made with calcium sulfate and magnesium chloride
Serving Size: ½ cup: firm vs soft
Calories: 88 / 76
Protein: 10.3 g / 8 g
Total Fat: 5.2 g / 4.6 g
Carbohydrates: 2 g / 2 g
Fiber: 1 g / 0 g
Cholesterol: 0 mg / 0 mg
Calcium: 253 mg, 25% DRI / 138 mg, 14% DRI
Iron: 2 mg, 15% DRI / 1.4 mg, 11% DRI
Magnesium: 47 mg, 12% DRI / 33 mg, 9% DRI

Health Benefits
Soybeans and the most common soybean product, tofu, are rich in plant protein and phytonutrients called isoflavones. Controversy continues about the estrogen-like effects of isoflavones

on women, especially women who are concerned about estrogen-related cancers. Research indicates that women should avoid processed soy products and supplements that contain isoflavones in purified forms, and instead chose whole soy foods such as soybeans, tofu, and whole soy flour.

- Isoflavones may reduce the risk of breast cancer by binding to estrogen receptor sites in the mammary gland cells. In this way, isoflavones are similar to the anticancer drug for breast cancer called tamoxifen. One isoflavone, called genistein, fights tumors by inhibiting the enzymes needed for their growth and reducing the blood supply which allows them to grow.
- Soy's ability to reduce cholesterol has been attributed, at least in part, to genistein. In fact, the Food and Drug Administration officially stated in 1999 that twenty-five grams of soy protein daily may reduce the risk of heart disease.
- A 2008 report in the *Expert Review of Anticancer Therapy* notes that soy is effective in reducing the risk of prostate cancer.
- Soy has shown promise in slowing bone loss in post-menopausal osteoporosis. More research is needed in this area.
- The ability of soy foods to reduce menopausal symptoms (e.g., hot flashes, night sweats) is uncertain, with some studies reporting significant success while others show no benefit.

How to Select and Store

Dried soybeans are usually available in bulk bins or in prepackaged containers. In either case, look for whole, non-cracked beans that have no sign of moisture. Soybeans are also available in cans. Fresh soybeans, or edamame, should be deep green and have firm, unblemished pods. Edamame is usually found in the frozen food section; some Asian markets may have them in the produce aisle.

Store dried soybeans in an airtight container in a dry, cool, dark place, where they should keep for up to twelve months. Once cooked, soybeans will keep fresh in the refrigerator for about three days if kept in a covered container. Fresh edamame should be refrigerated and eaten within two days. Frozen edamame will keep fresh for three to four months.

TOFU BURGERS
12 oz extra-firm tofu, crumbled or mashed
¾ cup quick rolled oats
½ tsp onion powder
2 Tbs soy sauce
½ tsp each: basil, oregano, garlic powder
Dash salt and pepper

Drain and crumble the tofu. Mix ingredients with the tofu, kneading for a few minutes by hand. Shape into tofu burger patties. Bake on a lightly greased baking sheet at 325° F for 20–25 minutes. Serve with your favorite toppings.

TOFU CORN CHOWDER
Serves 2
6 oz soft tofu
1 cup cream-style corn
1 cup water
1 cup red or green bell pepper, finely chopped
Salt and pepper to taste
Chopped green onions (optional)

In a blender, puree tofu with water, add the corn, and blend. Transfer to a pot, add the peppers, and heat until simmering, stirring occasionally. Add salt and pepper, and garnish with chopped onions if desired.

SPINACH

Spinach is part of the "greens" family, but it's such a power-house of nutrition it deserves to have its own entry. Experts believe spinach originated in ancient Persia, and then was transported to China in the seventh century and to Europe in the eleventh century. Catherine de Medici, who lived in the sixteenth century, loved spinach so much she always made sure she had cooks who could prepare it especially for her. The term "à la Florentine," which refers to any dish prepared on a bed of spinach, is attributed to her.

The largest commercial growers of spinach today are the United States and the Netherlands.

Spinach Nutrition
Serving Size: 1 cup cooked
Calories: 41
Protein: 5.4 g
Total Fat: 0.5 g
Carbohydrates: 6.8 g
Fiber: 4.3 g
Cholesterol: 0 mg
Vitamin A: 18,866 IU, 725% DRI
Vitamin K: 888 mcg, 846% AI
Calcium: 245 mg, 25% DRI
Iron: 6.43 mg, 49% DRI
Manganese: 1.68 mg, 84% DRI
Magnesium: 157 mg, 41% DRI

Health Benefits
Experts have identified at least thirteen different flavonoid compounds in spinach that provide antioxidant and/or anticancer benefits. These substances, along with other nutrients, offer a variety of healthy reasons to eat spinach—often!

- Spinach contains a carotenoid called neoxanthin, which research shows can cause prostate cancer cells to self-destruct.
- Vitamin K helps maintain bone health by activating osteocalcin, the major non-collagen protein in bone. Spinach also provides calcium and magnesium, which help prevent osteoporosis.

- Spinach is an excellent source of iron, which is critical for women in menopause and for people who have anemia or chronic fatigue syndrome.
- The lutein found in spinach helps protect against age-related macular degeneration and cataracts, as well as atherosclerosis. To boost the bioavailability of lutein in spinach, enjoy this green with olive oil and/or hard-boiled eggs.
- Inflammatory conditions—e.g., arthritis, asthma, bursitis, heart disease, migraine—may improve with help from the nutrients in spinach, including beta-carotene, vitamin C, magnesium, and riboflavin.
- The beta-carotene and vitamin C in spinach may help prevent atherosclerosis and diabetic heart disease by reducing free radicals and preventing the oxidation of cholesterol so it cannot stick to the walls of the blood vessels.
- Folate in spinach may help prevent the buildup of homocysteine, a substance that can lead to stroke or heart attack.
- The magnesium in spinach may reduce high blood pressure and protect against heart disease.
- Spinach contains vitamin E, which helps slow mental decline and memory loss.

How to Select and Store

Choose fresh spinach that has deep green, tender leaves. Avoid bunches that contain slimy leaves. Store fresh spinach loosely packed and unwashed in a plastic bag in the refrigerator, where it should stay fresh for four to five days.

GREEN JUICE
Serves 2
1 bunch each, organic: spinach, romaine lettuce, kale
3–4 organic apples
2–3 organic lemons

Wash the greens, peel the apples and lemons, and juice in a juicer. Chill and enjoy.

SPINACH LENTIL SOUP
Serves 1
½ cup lentils
1 cup almond milk
1 cup spinach
3 Tbs nutritional yeast flakes
1 tsp garlic powder
1 tsp cumin
¼ tsp cayenne pepper
Pinch salt

Place all ingredients into a pot and bring to a boil. Reduce heat and simmer until the lentils are done to your liking. Stir in the spinach and remove the pot from the heat.

SQUASH

The term "squash" includes vegetables that are members of the *Cucurbitaceae* family, and relatives of the cucumber and melon. Summer squash varieties include crookneck and straight neck squash, pattypan squash, and zucchini; the most common winter squash varieties are acorn, butternut, Hubbard, pumpkin, and spaghetti.

Modern-day squash developed from the wild squash that have been growing for more than ten thousand years in Central America and Mexico. Originally squash were cultivated for their seeds alone, because the vegetables did not have much flesh. Over time, various cultivation techniques resulted in fleshier, better-tasting varieties. Today the largest commercial producers of squash are China, Japan, Romania, Turkey, Italy, Egypt, and Argentina.

Squash Nutrition

Acorn Squash
Serving Size: 1 cup mashed, cooked
Calories: 83

Protein: 1.6 g
Total Fat: 0 g
Carbohydrates: 21.5 g
Fiber: 6.4 g
Cholesterol: 0 mg
Iron: 1.4 mg, 11% DRI
Potassium: 644 mg, 14% AI
Vitamin A: 632 IU, 24% DRI
Vitamin C: 16 mg, 20% DRI

Hubbard Squash

Serving Size: 1 cup mashed, cooked
Calories: 71
Protein: 3.5 g
Total Fat: 0.8 g
Carbohydrates: 15 g
Fiber: 6.8 g
Cholesterol: 0 mg
Potassium: 505 mg, 11% AI
Vitamin A: 9,452 IU, 363% DRI

Zucchini

Serving Size: 1 cup, with skin, cooked, slices
Calories: 36
Protein: 1 g
Total Fat: 0 g
Carbohydrates: 7 g
Fiber: 2.5 g
Cholesterol: 0 mg
Folate: 36 mcg,
Potassium: 455 mg, 10% AI
Vitamin A: 2,011 IU, 77% DRI
Vitamin C: 10 mg, 12% DRI

Health Benefits

Although winter squash have both a more diverse nutritional content and higher levels of many of the nutrients, all squash offer health benefits. We discuss a few of them here.

- Research published in *Public Health Nutrition* shows that squash extracts may help reduce symptoms of an enlarged prostate, especially when they are consumed along with other foods that contain phytonutrients.
- Pumpkin is a rich source of beta-cryptoxanthin, a carotenoid that may significantly reduce the risk of lung cancer. A study of more than sixty thousand adults found that those who ate the most cryptoxanthin-rich foods had a twenty-seven percent reduced risk of lung cancer.
- Winter squash are an especially rich source of beta-carotene, which may prevent oxidation of cholesterol and thus help reduce the risk of atherosclerosis, heart attack, and stroke. It can also reduce the risk of colon cancer by protecting the intestinal tract from the damage inflicted by cancer-causing toxins.
- The carotenoids in squash may help regulate blood sugar in people with diabetes, and help with insulin resistance.
- Beta-carotene's anti-inflammatory properties may reduce symptoms of arthritis, asthma, fibromyalgia, and other inflammatory conditions.
- The fiber in squash may help with regularity, and to prevent and treat constipation, diarrhea, diverticular disease, hemorrhoids, and irritable bowel syndrome.
- The potassium in squash may help to control high blood pressure.

How to Select and Store

When choosing squash, select those that are heavy for their size. Specifically for summer squash, look for vegetables that have shiny and firm, but not hard, rinds. Choose squash of average size, as very large ones may be fibrous and very small ones may lack flavor. At home, refrigerate unwashed squash in a plastic bag, where it should keep fresh for up to seven days.

If you buy winter squash, choose those that have dull, hard rinds. Depending on the variety, winter squash can be kept for one week or up to six months. Uncut winter squash keep best when stored at fifty to sixty F; once it is cut, cover the squash in plastic wrap and store in the refrigerator, where it will keep for only one to two days.

STUFFED ACORN SQUASH
Serves 4
2 large acorn squash
4 large apples, peeled, cored, and cut into ½" pieces
2 Tbs honey
½ cup raisins

Cut squash in half and clean out the seeds. Place in a hot oven (350 F) and bake for 20 minutes. In the meantime, mix the remaining ingredients in a bowl. Spoon the mixture into the squash halves and bake for an additional 30 minutes. Let stand 5 minutes before serving.

SUMMER SQUASH TREAT
Serves 4
1 lb zucchini, sliced
1 lb crookneck squash, sliced
1 green bell pepper, sliced
2 small tomatoes, peeled and cut into wedges
1 small yellow onion, peeled and sliced
1 clove garlic, chopped
2 Tbs olive oil
1 tsp dried basil
½ cup shredded low-fat cheese, your choice
Salt and pepper to taste

Place onion, garlic, squash, tomatoes, bell pepper, and oil into a skillet and sauté on high heat. Sprinkle with basil. When the vegetables are slightly browned, remove from heat and place mixture into a serving bowl. Add salt and pepper. Sprinkle with cheese and cover the bowl to allow the cheese to melt. Stir to distribute the cheese, and serve.

STRAWBERRIES

Strawberries are reportedly the most popular berry in the world, and for good reason: they are juicy, sweet, fragrant, easy to eat, and they look like little hearts. They also are a stellar source of vitamin C and some less common phytonutrients that possess healing qualities.

Wild strawberries have grown for millennia in temperate areas of the world. The ancient Romans enjoyed them, and during the Middle Ages people valued them for medicinal and dietary reasons. Up until the eighteenth century strawberries were tiny, but crossbreeding between a South American and a North American variety resulted in a hybrid strawberry that is large and sweet. Today the largest commercial producers of strawberries are the United States, Canada, France, Italy, Japan, Australia, and New Zealand.

Strawberry Nutrition
  Serving Size: 1 cup, sliced
  Calories: 53
  Protein: 1 g
  Total Fat: 0.5 g
  Carbohydrates: 13 g
  Fiber: 3.3 g
  Cholesterol: 0 mg
  Folate: 40 mcg, 10% DRI
  Vitamin C: 98 mg, 110% DRI

Health Benefits
  Strawberries are a source of various phytonutrients that offer many benefits. Here's a closer look.

- The anthocyanins are potent antioxidants that help protect the body's organs against cell damage.
- Strawberries contain anti-inflammatory agents that can reduce the activity of the enzyme cyclo-oxygenase, or COX. This is the same ability that ibuprofen and aspirin possess, yet strawberries can help relieve inflammation associated with asthma, atherosclerosis, arthritis, fibromyalgia, and other conditions without the drugs' side effects, especially intestinal bleeding.
- The phytonutrient ellagitannin in strawberries has been linked with reduced cancer rates. A study of more than a thousand elderly people found that those who ate the most strawberries were three times less likely to develop cancer than those who ate few or none.
- Strawberries may help prevent macular degeneration. Studies show that fruit—much more than vegetables—protects against this vision-robbing disease. Three servings of fruit daily are recommended to provide the necessary antioxidants and carotenoids.
- High doses of vitamin C protect against the inflammation of arthritis, while low vitamin C intake is associated with a threefold greater likelihood of developing the disease, according to a study of more than twenty thousand people published in the *Annals of the Rheumatic Diseases*.
- The combination of high vitamin C content and phytonutrients makes strawberries a good choice for preventing and fighting bacterial, viral, and fungal infections (e.g., bronchitis, colds, ear infections, flu, urinary tract infections, vaginitis).

How to Select and Store

Strawberries are highly perishable, so only purchase an amount that you can use within two to three days, or that you plan to freeze. Select berries that are firm, plump, and that have their green caps attached. If you buy packaged strawberries, make sure they are not tightly packed and there is no evidence of moisture or mold.

Strawberries should be refrigerated. Remove any moldy or damaged berries from the bunch before you refrigerate them. Berries can be placed unwashed in a container or spread out on a plate and covered with a paper towel and plastic wrap. Do not leave strawberries at room temperature or exposed to sunlight, as they will spoil rapidly.

To freeze strawberries, first wash them gently, pat dry, and arrange them on a flat pan. Place the pan in the freezer. Once the berries are frozen, transfer them to a plastic bag and return them to the freezer, where they should keep for up to one year. Frozen berries will retain more of their vitamin C content if they are left whole.

STRAWBERRY SMOOTHIE
Serves 2
1 cup nonfat milk
3 Tbs wheat germ
1 cup sliced strawberries
1 small, very ripe banana
4 ice cubes

Place all ingredients into a blender and process at high speed until smooth.

STRAWBERRY SALSA
Makes 1½ cups
1 cup coarsely chopped strawberries
1 Tbs orange juice
1 green onion, finely chopped
2 Tbs dried currants
2 Tbs red wine vinegar
1 tsp Dijon-style mustard

Combine all ingredients in a bowl and chill. Serve with fish, chicken, or tofu.

SWEET POTATOES

Relics of 10,000-year-old sweet potatoes have been found in Peruvian caves, so people have been enjoying these root vegetables for a very long time. Sweet potatoes have yellow or orange flesh, and the skin may be white, orange, yellow, red, or purple. In the United States, the terms "sweet potato" and "yam" are used interchangeably. The orange-colored, moist-fleshed vegetable that is usually called a yam is really a sweet potato that is grown in the south. True yams are an entirely different genus than the sweet potato; they also have rough, scaly skins and are very low in beta-carotene compared with sweet potatoes.

Christopher Columbus introduced sweet potatoes to Europe after his first trip to the New World in 1492. During the sixteenth century, farmers began to cultivate sweet potatoes in the southern United States. Sweet potatoes have become a popular food among Asian and Latin American cultures. The main commercial producers of sweet potatoes today include China, Indonesia, Vietnam, Japan, India, and Uganda.

Sweet Potato Nutrition

Serving Size: 1 large, baked in skin
Calories: 162
Protein: 3.6 g
Total Fat: 0.3 g
Carbohydrates: 37 g
Fiber: 6 g
Cholesterol: 0 mg
Iron: 1.3 mg, 10% DRI
Potassium: 855 mg, 18% DRI
Vitamin A: 34,592 IU, 1330% DRI
Vitamin C: 35 mg, 42% DRI

Health Benefits

One good thing about sweet potatoes (and there are many good things about them) is that they are naturally sweet and can easily be used as a nutritious, guilt-free dessert. There are many health benefits as well.

- Sweet potatoes have been called an antidiabetic food because they can help stabilize blood sugar levels and reduce insulin resistance. A high carotenoid level may explain these benefits.
- High levels of the antioxidants beta-carotene and vitamin C in sweet potatoes may help prevent atherosclerosis, diabetic heart disease, and colon cancer.
- The anti-inflammatory properties associated with beta-carotene also make sweet potatoes a good choice in the prevention and treatment of arthritis, asthma, fibromyalgia, and other inflammatory conditions.
- Since vitamin A/beta-carotene is critical for maintaining the immune system, sweet potatoes may help in the prevention and/or treatment of bronchitis, colds and flu, ear infections, eczema, gingivitis, herpes, psoriasis, ulcers, urinary tract infections, and vaginitis.

How to Select and Store

Choose sweet potatoes that are firm and without cracks or bruises. Do not purchase sweet potatoes that are in a refrigerated section of the market because cold has a negative effect on the taste. Store sweet potatoes loose (not in a bag) in a cool, dark, well-ventilated place, where they will keep fresh for up to ten days.

SWEET POTATO SALAD
Serves 4
1 lb sweet potatoes
1½ cup chopped celery
½ cup chopped onion
¼ cup dried cranberries
¼ cup chopped walnuts
2 Tbs lemon juice
2 Tbs olive oil
Salt to taste

Bake the sweet potatoes in a 400° F oven for 45–60 minutes until tender. Cool and peel. Cut into chunks and combine with the celery, onion, walnuts, and cranberries. Whisk together the lemon juice and olive oil. Toss the potato mixture with the dressing and add salt.

SWEET POTATO CAKES

Serves 6
4 large sweet potatoes
3 eggs
1½ tsp salt
⅛ tsp ground black pepper
⅛ tsp ground cumin (optional)
1 tsp oil

Cook the sweet potatoes in any preferred manner, peel, and mash well. In a bowl, whisk the eggs and seasonings. Add the mashed potatoes and mix well. Put the oil in a large skillet and put on medium heat. When hot, drop the potato mixture into the skillet in a size you choose. Flatten each cake and brown on both sides. Serve with maple syrup, nonfat sour cream, nonfat yogurt, or other favorite topping.

TEMPEH

When people hear that tempeh is made with a mold, some shudder and swear they won't touch it. That would be unfortunate, because tempeh, a fermented food made from cooked soybeans, is not only nutritious but quite delicious as well. Tempeh has been a favorite food and an important source of protein for people in Indonesia for about two thousand years. Shortly after the Dutch colonized Indonesia, they introduced tempeh to Europeans. In recent years it has gained popularity throughout the world.

Tempeh is made using controlled fermentation and a Rhizopus mold, often referred to as tempeh starter. The starter binds the soybeans into a compact cake that has a firm texture and a nutty flavor, and which allows it to be used as an ingredient in soups, salads, sandwiches, casseroles, spreads, and as an entrée.

Tempeh Nutrition
Serving Size: 4 oz
Calories: 223
Protein: 20.6 g
Total Fat: 13 g
Carbohydrates: 10.6 g
Fiber: 7 g
Cholesterol: 0 mg
Calcium: 108 mg, 11% DRI
Copper: 0.6 mg, 66% DRI
Magnesium: 87.5 mg, 22% DRI
Manganese: 1.45 mg. 73% DRI
Vitamin B-6: 0.23 mg, 15% DRI
Riboflavin: 0.4 mg, 33% DRI

Health Benefits
Someone once described tempeh as "looking like particle board," which is a highly unflattering description for this tasty, nutritious food. Tempeh is unusual among plant foods in that it is a complete protein; that is, it contains all the essential amino acids. It also contains many phytonutrients, such as isoflavones and soy saponins, and is a very good source of manganese, copper, magnesium, and riboflavin. Here are just a few of the benefits you can expect from tempeh.

- Tempeh is a high-protein food, which is critical for fighting fatigue, building muscle, and controlling blood sugar levels.
- Soy protein can reduce cholesterol levels, compared with protein from animal sources, which tends to raise them as animal protein also includes cholesterol and saturated fat.
- Both the fiber and digestive enzymes created during the fermentation process benefit digestion, which can help prevent and treat heartburn, irritable bowel syndrome, diverticular disease, constipation, and diarrhea.
- Magnesium is important in the prevention of cardio-vascular disease, including atherosclerosis, heart at-

tack, and stroke. Magnesium also is a factor in more than three hundred enzymatic reactions, including those involved in energy production and protein synthesis.

- Tempeh contains isoflavones, which act like very weak estrogens. Isoflavones may help relieve symptoms of PMS and menopause, such as hot flashes, night sweats, and headache.
- An isoflavone called genistein, present in tempeh and other soy foods, has been associated with a lower incidence of prostate cancer. Studies show that genistein may prevent proliferation of cancer cells in the prostate, as well as stimulate the natural death of abnormal (cancerous) cells.
- Several studies indicate that soy foods like tempeh may help reduce bone loss that typically occurs after menopause, thus helping to prevent osteoporosis.

How to Select and Store

Tempeh is available in the refrigerated or freezer section and, depending on the brand, may be plain soy or contain vegetables and/or grains. Select tempeh that has a thin whitish film. A few black or gray spots are normal, but do not buy tempeh that has yellow, pink, or blue coloration. Refrigerated tempeh can keep for up to ten days, and frozen tempeh will stay fresh for several months.

TEMPEH TACOS
Serves 4
2 Tbs olive oil
1 onion, diced
8 oz tempeh, sliced into ½-inch cubes
1 Tbs soy sauce
1 tsp cumin
¼ cup fresh chopped cilantro
Fillings for tacos (lettuce, tomato, sprouts, cheese, taco sauce)
Flour tortillas or taco shells

Sauté the onion in a skillet with the olive oil until the onion is soft. Add tempeh, soy sauce, and cumin. Cook for about 5 minutes, stirring frequently. Remove from heat and stir in the cilantro. Fill tortillas or taco shells with the tempeh mixture and favorite toppings.

TEMPEH STROGANOFF

Serves 4

8 oz five-grain tempeh, cut into ¼ inch cubes
4 Tbs margarine
2 onions, chopped
1 cup sliced mushrooms
2 cloves garlic, diced
2 Tbs soy sauce
1 cup vegetable bouillon
1 cup plain yogurt

Melt margarine in a skillet and sauté the onion and garlic until brown. Add the mushrooms, tempeh and soy sauce and sauté until the tempeh is browned. Add the bouillon, cover, and simmer 5 minutes. Remove from heat, add the yogurt, and stir. Serve over hot whole-grain noodles.

TOMATOES

A tomato is actually a fruit, not a vegetable. Tomatoes are believed to have originated on the western side of South America, including the Galapagos Islands. People in Mexico, however, first cultivated the plant. When the Spanish conquistadors went to Mexico around 1500, they brought tomato seeds back to Spain. By the sixteenth century tomatoes found their way to Italy, but because many people believed tomatoes were poisonous (the leaves are toxic), they did not become popular until later years. Tomatoes accompanied the colonists who settled in Virginia, but again it was some time before they became popular. Today, the major commercial producers of tomatoes are the United States, Russia, Italy, Spain, China, and Turkey.

Tomato Nutrition

Serving Size: 1 cup, red, chopped, raw
Calories: 32
Protein: 1.6 g
Total Fat: 0.4 g
Carbohydrates: 7 g
Fiber: 2.2 g
Cholesterol: 0 mg
Potassium: 427 mg, 9% AI
Vitamin A: 1,499 IU, 58% DRI
Vitamin C: 23 mg, 28% DRI

Serving Size: 1 cup, red, chopped, cooked
Calories: 43
Protein: 2.3 g
Total Fat: 0.3 g
Carbohydrates: 9.6 g
Fiber: 1.7 g
Cholesterol: 0 mg
Potassium: 523 mg, 11% AI
Vitamin A: 1,174 IU, 45% DRI
Vitamin C: 55 mg, 67% DRI

Health Benefits

Tomatoes have become synonymous with lycopene, the phytonutrient that protects against cancer in humans. A USDA Agricultural Research Service study found that lycopene levels were about three times greater in organic versus regular ketchup. Because this organic advantage probably applies to all tomato products, choose organic tomatoes and tomato products when possible.

• The consensus of a meta-analysis published in *Cancer Epidemiology Biomarkers and Prevention* is that men who ate the most raw tomatoes had an eleven percent reduction in risk for prostate cancer, while those who ate the most cooked tomatoes had a nineteen percent reduction.

- A three-year study published in the *Journal of Nutrition* reported that men who ate the most lycopene had a thirty-one percent reduction in the risk of pancreatic cancer.
- In the Women's Health Study, as the lycopene level rose in the nearly forty thousand women in the study, their risk of cardiovascular disease declined. After excluding women with angina, those with the highest lycopene levels had a fifty percent reduced risk of cardiovascular disease compared with women who had the lowest levels of lycopene.
- Tomatoes are a good source of vitamin K, which is necessary for bone health and the prevention of osteoporosis.
- The antioxidant and anti-inflammatory power of vitamin A and C in tomatoes may help ward off asthma, atherosclerosis, diabetic complications, heart disease, osteoporosis, and stroke.

How To Select and Store

Look for organic tomatoes that have a deep, rich color, which indicates a high level of lycopene. The skins should be smooth and without soft spots. Ripe tomatoes yield to slight pressure and smell sweet. To ripen tomatoes at home, keep them at room temperature and out of direct sunlight. To speed up ripening, place tomatoes in a paper bag with a banana or apple. You can slow the ripening process by placing tomatoes in the refrigerator. Ripe tomatoes typically keep for one to three days.

STUFFED BAKED TOMATOES
Serves 4
4 medium tomatoes, peeled
1 cup nonfat yogurt, plain
¼ cup chopped red onion
¼ cup chopped walnuts
4 tsp chopped fresh cilantro

Slice the stem end of the tomatoes. Use a sharp knife to make 3 or 4 vertical cuts onto the top of each tomato, cutting about halfway through the tomato. Place each tomato cut side up into an ungreased square baking dish. Pour ¼ inch of water into the dish. Preheat broiler. In a small bowl combine the yogurt and onion, spoon a heaping tablespoon of the mixture into each tomato. Broil for 4 minutes or until bubbly and light brown. Remove from the oven and garnish with walnuts and cilantro.

TOMATO SAUCE
Makes about 1 quart
¼ cup olive oil
1 ½ tsp crushed red pepper flakes
½ tsp salt
3 medium cloves garlic, minced
1 cup sliced mushrooms
1 28-oz can of crushed red tomatoes
Zest of one lemon

Combine the olive oil, red pepper flakes, salt, mushrooms, and garlic in a saucepan. Sauté for about 1 minute; do not let the garlic brown. Stir in the tomatoes and heat to a gentle simmer. Remove from heat and taste; add salt and/or pepper as needed. Stir in the lemon zest.

TUNA

Tuna is one of the most popular food fish in the world and, for many people, it is the only fish they will eat. It is available fresh, smoked, and canned, and the latter is the form most purchased in the United States. Fresh tuna, however, is a better source of the beneficial omega-3 fatty acids for which tuna is well known.

There are several varieties of tuna, including albacore (pale pink), bluefin (deep red), and yellowfin (also deep red).

Tuna is found in the warm-water regions of the Atlantic, Indian, and Pacific oceans, and in the Mediterranean Sea.

Tuna Nutrition
Serving Size for all: 3 oz

Yellowfin, cooked
Calories: 118
Protein: 25 g
Total Fat: 1 g
Carbohydrates: 0 g
Fiber: 0 g
Cholesterol: 49 mg
Niacin: 10 mg, 66% DRI
Selenium: 40 mcg, 73% DRI
Vitamin B-12: 0.5 mcg, 21% DRI
Vitamin B-6: 0.9 mg, 60% DRI

Bluefin, cooked
Calories: 156
Protein: 25 g
Total Fat: 5.3 g
Carbohydrates: 0 g
Fiber: 0 g
Cholesterol: 42 mg
Niacin:9 mg, 60% DRI
Selenium: 39 mcg, 71% DRI
Vitamin B-6: 0.4 mg, 27% DRI
Vitamin B-12: 9.25 mcg, 385% DRI

White, canned in water
Calories: 109
Protein: 20 g
Total Fat: 2.5 g
Carbohydrates: 0 g
Fiber: 0 g
Cholesterol: 36 mg
Niacin: 5 mg, 33% DRI

Selenium: 56 mcg, 100% DRI
Vitamin B-6: 0.2 mg, 13% DRI
Vitamin B-12: 1 mcg, 41% DRI

Health Benefits

Tuna is a very nutrient-dense food, and a great source of omega-3 fatty acids, protein, selenium, several B vitamins, and especially vitamin B-6, and it's low in fat. What does all this mean to you?

- Omega-3 fatty acids are heart-friendly: they help prevent and treat high blood pressure, heart attack, and heart disease, which they do by preventing blood clots, improving the ratio of good cholesterol to bad (high-density to low-density lipoproteins), and reducing inflammation.
- Tuna is a good source of vitamin B-6. This vitamin, along with folic acid, reduces levels of the harmful amino acid homocysteine, which in turn is an important risk factor for atherosclerosis.
- Tuna contains anti-inflammatory substances called resolvins, which inhibit the production and controls the movement of inflammatory cells to inflamed areas of the body, such as the joints in arthritis or blood vessel walls in atherosclerosis.
- A 2006 study found that children ages eight to thirteen years who increased their consumption of fish, including tuna, reduced their risk of developing asthma by about sixty-six percent.
- A study of more than ten thousand cancer patients who had nineteen different types of cancer found that eating small amounts of fish may protect against certain cancers, including ovarian, mouth, pharyngeal, esophageal, stomach, and colorectal cancer. A separate study found a thirty-seven percent reduced risk of colorectal cancer among people whose diets contained the most omega-3s compared with those who had the least. Animal and culture studies suggest that fish rich

in omega-3 fatty acids may protect against breast cancer, according to an *International Journal of Cancer* report.

How to Select and Store

When buying fresh tuna, smell it: fresh fish has only a slightly fishy smell, so do not buy tuna that has a strong fishy odor. Fresh, whole tuna should be displayed buried in ice, while steaks and fillets should be shown on top of ice.

Once you buy fresh tuna, refrigerate it as soon as possible because it is very sensitive to temperature. If you are transporting it in a car, place it in a cooler to keep it cold. To store fresh tuna at home, place the wrapped fish in a baking dish filled with ice and put the dish in the bottom shelf of the refrigerator. Replenish the ice one or two times daily. Refrigerated tuna can stay fresh for about four days if it was just caught before you bought it, or for one to two days if it was caught several days earlier. Freeze fresh tuna by wrapping it in plastic and placing in the coldest part of the freezer. It will keep for two to three weeks.

Canned tuna is packaged in broth, water, or oil. Because oil is high in omega-6 fatty acids (which promote inflammation), it is best to buy tuna packed in water or broth.

ZESTY LIME TUNA
Serves 4
4 tuna steaks, about 6 oz each
Zest and juice of one lime
2 tsp dried thyme
1 tsp coarsely ground black pepper
¼ tsp salt
2 tsp virgin olive oil

Rinse the tuna steaks and pat dry with paper towels. Grate the zest from the lime; squeeze the juice and set aside. In a small bowl, combine zest, thyme, pepper, and salt. Lightly rub the seasoning mixture on the tuna steaks, coating them well. In a heavy-bottomed pan, warm the oil, raise the heat to high and place the tuna in the pan. Sear for 1 minute, then turn over, reducing the heat to medium. Sear the other side for 1 minute until medium rare. Pour the lime juice over the tuna and serve immediately.

TUNA PITA
Serves 1
1 whole wheat pita
3 oz canned tuna, drained
2 Tbs chopped bell pepper
2 Tbs chopped red onion
1 Tbs nonfat yogurt
1 Tbs orange juice
½ cup shredded lettuce or sprouts

Combine tuna, bell pepper, onion, yogurt, and orange juice and mix well. Cut the pita, stuff it with the tuna mixture, and add lettuce or sprouts.

TURKEY

Although wild turkeys still populate the United States, most people are more familiar with domesticated turkeys. Turkeys are indigenous to the Americas and were domesticated around 10 BC by the Aztecs. The fowl was a staple food of the native peoples of Central and South America by the time European explorers arrived in the Americas. Columbus brought samples of turkey back to Spain, and the meat soon became popular in Europe. Today demand for turkey is much greater in the United States than in Europe.

Domesticated turkeys available in supermarkets today are very different from wild turkeys because they are artificially fed and bred to increase production and profits. The result is birds that cannot fly or breed naturally (they are too heavy to do either), and that must be injected with vegetable oil because the meat is too dry due to the artificial means by which they are produced.

Turkey Nutrition

Serving size: 4 oz dark meat only, roasted
Calories: 207
Protein: 32 g
Total Fat: 8 g
Carbohydrates: 0 g
Fiber: 0 g
Cholesterol: 77 mg
Iron: 1.5 mg, 11% DRI
Niacin: 7.5 mg, 53% DRI
Riboflavin: 0.3 mg, 25% DRI
Vitamin B-6: 0.6 mg, 40% DRI
Zinc: 2.3 mg, 26% DRI

Health Benefits

Turkey (without the skin) is lower in fat than most other meat, high in protein, and is a relatively good source of several essential nutrients. Here are a few benefits that turkey may offer.

- Turkey is a good source of iron, which can benefit those who suffer with anemia and/or with fatigue associated with chronic fatigue syndrome, arthritis, fibromyalgia, or other disorders.
- The amino acid trytophan is abundant in turkey, and it is helpful for people who have sleep difficulties, including insomnia. Eating a small portion of turkey before bedtime may help with sleep.
- Turkey is a good source of zinc, which may be helpful for men who are experiencing erectile dysfunction.
- People who are overweight or obese may find turkey to be a good low-fat, high-protein alternative to other meat sources.
- Turkey provides healthy amounts of vitamin B-6 and zinc, which help reduce blood cholesterol, protect against cancer and heart disease, enhance nerve function, boost the immune system, and control blood pressure.

How to Select and Store

Choose organic turkey when possible. If you buy a fresh turkey, refrigerate it at 40° F or lower immediately when you get home, and use it within one to two days. To store leftover cooked turkey, refrigerate or freeze it within two hours of serving it. If the turkey was stuffed, remove the stuffing as soon as you take the turkey out of the oven and keep the stuffing separate from the meat. Leftover turkey will keep in the refrigerator for three to four days; stuffing should be used within one or two days. Frozen turkey should be eaten within one to two months.

TURKEY CHILI
Serves 6
½ cup each: chopped green, red, and yellow bell pepper
1 cup chopped onion
2 cloves garlic, minced
3 Tbs olive oil
2 cans kidney beans (15-oz cans)
2 cans stewed tomatoes, crushed (14-oz cans)
½ cup red wine
½ cup vegetable broth
3 cups cooked turkey, cut into ½-inch cubes
1 Tbs chili powder
1 Tbs chopped cilantro, fresh
½ tsp crushed red pepper flakes

In a large saucepan, sauté the peppers, onion, and garlic in oil until they are tender. Add the beans, tomatoes, wine, broth, turkey, chili powder, cilantro, and red pepper flakes. Bring to a boil; reduce heat to low and simmer, uncovered, for 25 minutes.

TURKEY SPRING SALAD
Serves 4
2 cups cooked turkey, chopped
1 small can water chestnuts, drained and diced
½ lb seedless green grapes, halved
½ cup chopped celery

½ cup slivered almonds
½ cup plain soy yogurt
1½ tsp curry powder
1 Tbs soy sauce
1 cup fresh pineapple, chopped
Lettuce leaves

Combine the turkey, water chestnuts, grapes, celery, and half
of the almonds. In a separate bowl, blend the yogurt with the
curry and soy sauce, then fold in the turkey mixture. Chill for
several hours, then serve on lettuce garnished with the remaining almonds and pineapple.

TURMERIC

Turmeric is a much revered spice/herb that comes from the
root of the *Curcuma longa* plant. Both Chinese and Ayurvedic
medicine practitioners have used turmeric for millennia for its
anti-inflammatory properties.

For more than 5,000 years, turmeric has been harvested in
its native regions of southern India and Indonesia. It is only
recently that it has gained popularity in Western cultures,
partly because research has highlighted its healing properties.
If you buy turmeric, it most likely will have been produced
in one of its native countries or in China, the Philippines,
Taiwan, Haiti, or Jamaica.

Turmeric Nutrition
   Serving Size: 1 tsp ground
   Calories: 8
   Protein: 0 g
   Total Fat: 0 g
   Carbohydrates: 1.4 g
   Fiber: 0.5 g
   Cholesterol: 0 mg

Health Benefits

You won't see a list of vitamins and minerals associated with turmeric, but its healing properties come in other forms. Many of the health benefits offered by turmeric appear to be linked to its volatile oil and, more importantly, to its orange or yellow pigment, called curcumin.

- The anti-inflammatory effects of curcumin can relieve the inflammation and pain associated with arthritis, bursitis, fibromyalgia, and tendonitis. Studies show that curcumin's anti-inflammatory effects compare with those of over-the-counter (e.g., ibuprofen) and prescription medications (e.g., hydrocortisone, phenylbutazone), but without the side effects.
- Curcumin may be effective in the treatment of intestinal disorders, including Crohn's disease and ulcerative colitis.
- Curcumin has the ability to help destroy mutated cancer cells, thus inhibiting the spread of cancer. This is especially important in the colon, where cell turnover occurs approximately every three days and the opportunity for cancer to spread is high.
- Studies show that frequent use of turmeric results in lower rates of breast, colon, lung, and prostate cancer.
- Bisdemethoxycurcumin, the most active ingredient in turmeric root, enhances the activity of the immune system in Alzheimer's disease.
- Curcumin helps lower cholesterol by instructing liver cells to increase the production of proteins (mRNA messenger proteins) which in turn help create receptors for bad (LDL) cholesterol. The addition of LDL receptors allows the liver to eliminate more LDL cholesterol from the body.

How to Select and Store

To get the best concentration of curcumin (the most active and potent part of turmeric), buy pure turmeric powder rather than curry powder. Turmeric powder should be stored in a tightly sealed container and kept in a cool, dry, dark place. Do not refrigerate: humidity will destroy turmeric.

TIPS ON USING TURMERIC

Turmeric is best known for its use in curried dishes, but it can enhance many other foods as well. Here are a few tips on how to use turmeric.

- Enhance your salad dressing by adding a teaspoon of turmeric powder and shaking well.
- Sprinkle a generous amount of turmeric (and some olive oil, depending on the recipe) on steamed vegetables.
- Combine a heaping teaspoon of ground turmeric and a teaspoon or two of olive oil. Steam your favorite vegetables—bite-size pieces of cauliflower, broccoli, bell pepper strips, carrot strips, squash, mushrooms— remove from heat, and drizzle the olive oil mixture on them. Add salt and pepper to taste if desired.
- Stir turmeric into existing condiments, such as mayonnaise, sour cream, and ketchup.
- Add turmeric to the water when making brown rice: 1 teaspoon of turmeric per 1 cup of uncooked rice.

TURNIPS

Some people turn their nose up at turnips, which were once considered a poor man's food, but these cruciferous root vegetables contain a long list of disease-preventing phytonutrients. Turnips originated in western Asia, and were used as food for both people and animals for millennia. When turnips were introduced to Europe, they were considered a staple food before potatoes eventually edged them out. Jacques Cartier brought turnips to the New World and planted them in Canada in 1541. Colonists in Virginia planted turnips in 1609, and the Native Americans soon adopted them as well.

Turnips come in various sizes and shapes, but the most common have white skin with shades of purple, green, or red-pink. Today, turnips are grown primarily in Asia, Europe, and in the northern United States and Canada.

Turnip Nutrition
Serving Size: 1 cup mashed
Calories: 51
Protein: 1.6 g
Total Fat: 0 g
Carbohydrates: 11.6 g
Fiber: 4.6 g
Cholesterol: 0 mg
Vitamin B-6: 0.15 mg, 10% DRI
Vitamin C: 27 mg, 33% DRI

Health Benefits
Turnips are an often neglected vegetable that is high in vitamin C (turnip juice has twice the amount of vitamin C as orange juice) and many phytonutrients. Traditional Chinese and Asian medicine has long held that eating turnips improves circulation and helps clear respiratory problems such as bronchitis, asthma, and cough. Let's see what the research says.

- Turnips contain very high levels of phytonutrients called glucosinolates, which are responsible for the secretion of special enzymes that remove cancer-causing substances from the body.
- The high fiber in turnips promotes regularity and helps prevent and treat intestinal conditions, including colorectal cancer, constipation, diarrhea, diverticular diseases, hemorrhoids, and irritable bowel syndrome.
- Turnips provide a healthy dose of vitamin C, a potent antioxidant that boosts the immune system and may help prevent or treat infections ranging from the common cold to ear infections, flu, gingivitis, herpes, urinary tract infections, and vaginitis.

How to Select and Store

When buying turnips, choose those that are heavy for their size and that have smooth skin. Smaller turnips are sweeter than larger ones. If you buy turnips with their tops attached, remove the greens before storing the roots. Refrigerated turnips usually stay fresh in the crisper for several weeks or for up to four months in a root cellar.

TANGY TURNIPS

Serves 4–6

2 lbs turnips
¼ tsp salt
¼ cup orange juice
½ tsp grated ginger
¼ tsp orange zest
1 Tbs margarine

Remove the turnip greens and set aside. Remove the crown of the turnips with a sharp knife. Peel the turnips and cut into 1-inch cubes. Steam the cubes until tender, drain, and mash. Using a whisk, beat all the remaining ingredients with the turnips until well mixed. Put the turnip mixture into a glass baking dish and bake at 350° F for 6–8 minutes.

TURMERIC TURNIPS

Serves 4–6

4 turnips, peeled and sliced
2 cups celery, chopped
4 tomatoes, sliced
2½ cups water
½ cup red wine
2 Tbs olive oil
1 tsp ground turmeric (or more, to taste)

Place all ingredients in a large covered pot and simmer for 25–30 minutes, stirring occasionally.

VEGETABLE JUICE

Tomato-based vegetable juice is a popular, nutritious beverage that can be enjoyed any time of the day. Although the amount and number of nutrients vary based on which brand and variety of vegetable juice you buy (some have added antioxidants and/or calcium, for example), 100% vegetable juices that have a tomato base generally offer a similar core of nutrients (see below).

One advantage of 100% vegetable juice products is that they allow people to get a substantial amount of their daily recommended intake of vegetables in a convenient, delicious way. Vegetable juices can be consumed in your car, at home, on a train, any time of the day, and they are a great way to end a meal, especially if you didn't eat your veggies.

Vegetable Juice Nutrition

Serving Size: 8 oz, commercial brand 100% vegetable juice (check your favorite brand for its nutritional content)
Calories: 49
Protein: 2 g
Total Fat: 0 g
Carbohydrates: 10 g
Fiber: 2 g
Cholesterol: 0 mg
Potassium: 469 mg, 10% DRI
Vitamin A: 2,000 IU, 76% DRI
Vitamin C: 30 mg, 36% DRI

Health Benefits

Drink to your health with 100% vegetable juice. One advantage is that you can add more nutritious ingredients to this basic, already-nutritious juice. For example, a teaspoon of turmeric, a tablespoon of flaxseed or flaxseed oil, or another vegetable juice, such as carrot, can contribute a powerful punch. Of course, vegetable juice alone is great as well.

- Tomato-based vegetable juice contains lycopene, a phytonutrient that is credited with helping reduce the development of prostate cancer and cancers of the digestive tract. Research shows that processed tomato products—such as vegetable juice—have a much greater level of lycopene than raw tomatoes.
- Lycopene may reduce the risk of macular degeneration and the development of cancer of the bladder, cervix, lung, and skin.
- A *Journal of Nutrition* article reports that women with the highest intake of tomato-based foods, including vegetable juice, had a significantly reduced risk for cardiovascular disease compared to women with a low intake. Women who ate seven or more servings of tomato-based foods per week had a thirty percent reduction in risk; those who ate ten or more had a sixty-five percent reduced risk for conditions such as stroke and heart attack.
- The combination of vitamins A and C plus lycopene makes vegetable juice a good choice to prevent and treat eye conditions, including cataracts, glaucoma, and macular degeneration, as well as promote overall eye health.
- The high vitamin A/beta-carotene content in vegetable juice may help prevent and treat acne, bursitis, colds and flu, constipation, ear infections, eczema, gingivitis, herpes, psoriasis, ulcers, and urinary tract infections.
- A 2007 study found that foods rich in vitamin A and lycopene may relieve symptoms of asthma.

How to Select and Store

There are several brands of 100% vegetable juice, and each offers one or more varieties; for example, added antioxidants, added calcium, spicy, low sodium, and/or organic. If possible, choose an organic variety to get optimal nutritional value. Once opened, refrigerate the juice and use it within five to seven days.

GAZPACHO

Serves 6
6 tomatoes, peeled and chopped
1½ cups vegetable juice
1 medium cucumber, peeled and chopped
1 medium onion, finely diced
1 small bell pepper, finely diced
2 cloves garlic, minced
¼ cup olive oil
2 Tbs vinegar
Hot sauce to taste

Combine all ingredients in a large bowl and chill for several
hours before serving.

SOUTHWEST KICKER

Serves 6
4 cups vegetable juice
⅛ tsp cayenne powder
⅛ tsp cumin powder
⅛ tsp turmeric powder
Lime slices for garnish

Combine the juice with the spices, shake well, and garnish
with lime.

WALNUTS

The walnut is a popular tree nut that has been cultivated for
millennia and prized as a food, medicine, and dye, and for its
oil for lamps. The oldest archaeological evidence of walnuts
was found in a cave in northern Persia (Iraq). Romans introduced the walnut to Europe in the fourth century AD, and it
has been grown there ever since. The English walnut originated in India. White and black walnuts are native to North
America and were popular with Native Americans as well as
the early colonists. Today, California produces nearly one

hundred percent of the walnuts consumed in the United States, and two-thirds of the world's supply. Other major commercial producers of walnuts are China, France, Romania, Iran, and Turkey.

Walnut Nutrition
Serving Size: 1 oz
Calories: 185
Protein: 4.3 g
Total Fat: 18.5 g
Carbohydrates: 3.9 g
Fiber: 2 g
Cholesterol: 0 mg
Manganese: 0.9 mg, 42% DRI
Copper: 0.45 mg, 50% DRI

Health Benefits
Walnuts have been getting very positive press when it comes to health benefits. Although they are high in fat, most of the fat is "good" fat: less than ten percent is saturated. With all their advantages, it appears walnuts should be kept on the "must have" grocery list.

- Results from the Nurses' Health Study show that women who eat at least one ounce of nuts or peanuts per week have a twenty-five percent lower risk of developing gallstones.
- Monounsaturated fats can help reduce high cholesterol levels and other risks for cardiovascular disease. Research shows that people who followed a diet rich in monounsaturated fats (thirty-five percent of which came from walnuts) had lower levels of cholesterol than people who did not follow the diet.
- The omega-3 fatty acids in walnuts may reduce the tendency for blood clots (and lower the risk of stroke and heart attack), improve cholesterol levels, and reduce inflammation.

- Omega-3 fatty acids also promote bone health because they prevent excessive turnover of bone and thus help prevent osteoporosis.
- Walnuts contain high levels of the amino acid L-arginine, which is a major player in controlling high blood pressure. That's because L-arginine is converted into nitric oxide, a chemical that helps blood vessels to relax and thus facilitates blood flow.
- An antioxidant called ellagic acid, which is present in walnuts, may block the processes that can lead to cancer. Ellagic acid can also protect healthy cells from free-radical damage and prevent cancer cells from reproducing.

How to Select and Store

If you buy whole, unshelled walnuts, choose ones that feel heavy for their size and that are not cracked or stained. Shelled walnuts should look plump and smell fresh (sniff them if you are buying from a bulk bin). Store shelled walnuts in an airtight container and refrigerate them; they should keep fresh for up to six months. Frozen shelled walnuts should last up to one year. Unshelled walnuts should be refrigerated but can be kept in a cool, dark, dry place for up to six months.

WALNUT COLESLAW
Serves 6
1 cup walnuts, coarsely chopped
1 cup dried cranberries
2 cups red cabbage, finely sliced
2 cups green cabbage, finely sliced
¼ cup thinly sliced red onion
Dressing: ⅓ cup each: cider vinegar, olive oil, sugar
1 tsp celery seed

Combine all the vegetables in a large bowl. Place all the dressing ingredients into a shaker bottle and shake well. Pour dressing over vegetables, mix well, and chill for at least 3 hours before serving. Before serving, mix well and then drain off any excess dressing (if desired).

MERRY WALNUTS
Makes 2 cups
2 cups shelled whole walnuts
2½ Tbs olive oil
2 tsp crumbled dried rosemary
1½ tsp salt
½ tsp cayenne pepper

Preheat oven to 350° F. Place walnuts in a single layer in a shallow pan. Mix together the remaining ingredients and drizzle over the nuts. Roast in oven for 10 minutes, shaking occasionally.

WATER

Water is essential for life, and the quality of the water you consume can have a dramatic impact on your health. If you have ever gotten a case of "traveler's diarrhea" after drinking water in a country or region that does not have adequate water treatment, you know what we mean.

The human body is fifty to sixty percent water, depending on your gender (men have a higher percentage) and body type. The body loses water every day in urine, feces, sweat, and breath, and it must be replaced daily to maintain health. Even mild dehydration—a drop of only one to two percent in body weight—can result in significant symptoms, including dizziness, fatigue, headache, and muscle weakness. People can live only ten to fourteen days without water.

Water Nutrition
Water has no calories or macronutrients, but it does contain minerals. "Hard" water contains dissolved minerals such as calcium and magnesium, which are the most common; aluminum, iron, and/or manganese are present in some water

supplies. "Soft" water has been treated to remove minerals but contains sodium (salt). The amount of minerals and sodium in hard and soft water varies according to the supplier, region, and how it is treated. Some people install water softeners in their homes to remove the minerals from their water.

Health Benefits

Sufficient amounts of water are essential for virtually every process in the human body. Space does not permit us to list all the health benefits you get from consuming a sufficient amount of pure water. Here are just a few:

- Your energy level is determined largely by the amount of water you consume. A five percent drop in body fluids, for example, will result in a twenty-five to thirty percent decline in energy in most people.
- Drinking enough water and other fluids helps to keep dissolved minerals from forming into stones in the kidneys.
- A two percent decline in body water can cause short-term memory difficulties.
- Drinking sufficient water helps reduce constipation and helps promote regularity.
- Research shows that drinking sufficient amounts of water daily decreases the risk of colon cancer by forty-five percent and bladder cancer by fifty percent.
- Drinking water helps you feel full and is an aid to losing weight.
- Preliminary research indicates that drinking eight to ten glasses of water daily could reduce joint and back pain for as many as eighty percent of people who suffer with these problems.

How to Select and Store

To ensure you have the best drinking water possible, you can check with your municipal water supplier and ask for the annual water quality report. Based on the substances that are present in your municipal water supply, you may want to choose a water

filtration system to eliminate some of these substances. To help
you select a water filtration system that addresses your specific
needs, you can check with the Water Quality Association, a
nonprofit international organization that represents the water
treatment industry for consumers and businesses. See http://
www.wqa.org

WATERCRESS

Although it doesn't get much attention, watercress (*Nasturtium officinale*) is one of the healthiest vegetables you can eat.
This member of the cruciferous family, and native plant of
Europe and Asia, can be traced back to the Persians, Romans,
and Greeks, who recognized that this green vegetable improved growth, strength, and stamina. Centuries ago watercress was the first food people turned to when wheat was
scarce. It was also known as scurvy grass, because it is rich
with the nutrients that can prevent this disease. Hippocrates so
revered this plant that he is said to have chosen the location of
his first hospital because it was close to fresh watercress,
which he used to treat patients.

Watercress has a distinctly pepper or mustard taste. It is
very popular in Great Britain, where there is a society dedi-
cated to promoting and preserving it. The eastern United
States, however, is the world's largest producer of watercress.

Watercress Nutrition
  Serving Size: 1 cup chopped
  Calories: 4
  Protein: 0.8 g
  Total Fat: 0 g
  Carbohydrates: 0.4 g
  Fiber: 0.2 g
  Cholesterol: 0 mg
  Thiamin: 0.3 mg, 22 % DRI
  Vitamin A: 1085 IU, 42% DRI

Vitamin B-6: 0.4 mg, 26% DRI
Vitamin C: 15 mg, 18% DRI
Vitamin K: 85 mcg, 80% AI

Health Benefits

According to folklore, watercress can treat everything from colds to diabetes, indigestion, gallstones, and cancer. The Chinese have long honored its use as a detoxifier. Scientists have found evidence that watercress is indeed beneficial for many health problems. These advantages are associated with the high levels of vitamins and phytonutrients in the plant. What does the research show?

- A double-blind, placebo-controlled study of a watercress extract found it to be effective in preventing recurrent urinary tract infections, as reported in *Current Medical Research and Opinion*.
- A University of Ulster study reported that eating watercress daily (eighty-five grams) can significantly reduce DNA damage to blood cells, which is linked to the development of cancer, plus boost the ability to the cells to ward off further DNA damage caused by free radicals. These benefits were most evident in smokers.
- Watercress is rich in the flavonoid quercetin, which reduces inflammation and is a natural antihistamine. Thus watercress may help prevent and treat allergies, asthma, colds, and sinusitis. The German Commission E recognizes watercress as an effective treatment for respiratory conditions.
- Preliminary studies suggest quercetin may be effective in the treatment of prostatitis (enlarged prostate).
- In China, watercress is eaten to treat gingivitis.
- Watercress is a very good source of beta-carotene, lutein, and zeaxanthin, which promote healthy skin and eyes, and may help prevent and treat acne, cataracts, eczema, glaucoma, macular degeneration, and psoriasis.

How to Select and Store

Look for bright green, perky leaves. To store watercress, place the bunch in a container of water, as you would a bouquet of flowers. Loosely cover the top with plastic, and it should stay fresh in the refrigerator for up to five days.

WATERCRESS SOUP
Serves 6
3 4-inch pieces of dried wakame
1 cup sliced onion
6 cups water
1 ½ Tbs miso
½ cup chopped scallions
½ oz parsley
3 bunches watercress, chopped into 3-inch pieces

Rinse the wakame and slice it into ½-inch pieces. Put the wakame and onions into a pot and add the water. Bring to a boil, reduce the heat and simmer 10–20 minutes. Reduce to very low heat. Place the miso in a bowl, add ½ cup of the broth from the pot, and puree until the miso is completely dissolved. Add the pureed miso to the soup, along with the watercress, scallions, parsley, and ginger. Simmer 3–5 minutes.

STIR-FRY WATERCRESS
Serves 4
2 Tbs soy sauce
1 Tbs miso
1 Tbs rice vinegar
2 Tbs sliced almonds
6 bunches watercress, cut into 2–4-inch pieces
2 Tbs sesame oil
1 Tbs fresh ginger, finely chopped

Combine the soy sauce, miso, and vinegar until smooth. Heat a wok and stir-fry the almonds until toasted. Remove the almonds from the wok. Add the sesame oil to the wok and heat.

When hot, add watercress and ginger and stir-fry until tender, about 2–3 minutes. Drizzle the miso dressing over the watercress and serve.

WATERMELON

Hieroglyphics provide evidence that watermelons were cultivated by the ancient Egyptians. In fact, the Egyptians so highly regarded watermelons, they placed them in the tombs of their kings. In the tenth century watermelons were introduced to China, and they later made their way throughout the western hemisphere. Today, the Russians make a popular wine from watermelon, and that country is a major producer of watermelons, as are China, Turkey, Iran, and the United States. In the United States alone, producers grow more than two hundred varieties of watermelon.

Watermelon Nutrition
Serving Size: 1 cup balls/diced
Calories: 46
Protein: 1 g
Total Fat: 0 g
Carbohydrates: 12 g
Fiber: 1 g
Cholesterol: 0 mg
Vitamin A: 556 IU, 21% DRI
Vitamin C: 14.5 mg, 17% DRI

Health Benefits
To get the most nutrition from a watermelon, eat it when it is fully ripe. That's when its antioxidants and other nutrients are at their peak.

• Watermelon is a good source of vitamins A (beta-carotene) and C, which may reduce the risk of heart disease and colon cancer, as well as relieve symptoms of arthritis and asthma.

- Watermelon has exceptionally high levels of citrulline, an amino acid used to make arginine (another amino acid), which can play a key role in treating erectile dysfunction, high blood pressure, insulin sensitivity, and atherosclerosis.
- The lycopene in watermelon may significantly reduce the risk of developing prostate cancer. In a study involving 130 men who had prostate cancer and 274 controls, men who consumed the most fruits and vegetables rich in lycopene (e.g., watermelon, papaya, tomatoes, guava) were 82 percent less likely to develop prostate cancer compared with men who ate the least amount of lycopene-rich foods.

How to Select and Store

When choosing a cut watermelon, look for pulp that has a deep color and no white streaks. If it is a seeded melon, the seeds should be deep in color. If you are buying a whole melon, it should be heavy for its size and have a relatively smooth rind that isn't too shiny or too dull. One side of the melon should have an area that is yellowish or creamy in color, which indicates that it was allowed to ripen on the ground and was likely harvested at the right time.

Store your melon at room temperature, because the quality of carotenoids (e.g., lycopene, beta-carotene) increases. Once a watermelon is cut, however, you should refrigerate it to retain its juiciness, freshness, and taste. Cover cut parts of the melon with plastic wrap to prevent drying.

WATERMELON LASAGNA
Serves 6
4 cups whole wheat or bran flakes
2 cups minced watermelon
2 cups sliced strawberries or whole blueberries
2 cups low-fat soy vanilla yogurt

Place ⅓ of the cereal in an even layer in the bottom of an 8 × 8 serving dish. Mix the fruit with the yogurt and spoon half of it over the flakes. Sprinkle ⅓ of the flakes over the yogurt and then spoon the remaining yogurt onto the second layer of chips. Sprinkle the remaining flakes on top and chill.

WATERMELON CRUNCH
Serves 6
4 cups watermelon balls
4 oz low-fat cream cheese
½ cup low-fat vanilla soy yogurt
¼ cup diced red bell pepper
1 ¼ cups diced celery
½ cup pecans

Blend the cream cheese with the yogurt, then stir in the celery and bell pepper. Place watermelon balls in dessert glasses and spoon the yogurt mixture on top. Sprinkle with pecans.

WHEAT GERM

At the very center of a wheat kernel (berry) is the germ, the part of the seed that is responsible for the growth and development of the wheat plant. Wheat germ is a highly concentrated source of protein, fiber, and various vitamins and minerals—twenty-three nutrients in all—and thus is one of the most nutritious foods you can eat.

Wheat germ has been described as tasting like straw, but toasting the germ brings out its nutty flavor and also helps keep it fresher longer. Both untoasted and toasted wheat germ are available in stores; untoasted wheat germ can easily be toasted in the oven.

Wheat Germ Nutrition
Serving Size: ¼ cup
Calories: 103
Protein: 6.5 g
Total Fat: 3.8 g
Carbohydrates: 15 g

Fiber: 3.7 g
Cholesterol: 0 mg
Iron: 1.8 mg, 14% DRI
Folate: 80 mcg, 20% DRI
Selenium: 22.7 mg, 40% DRI
Thiamin: 0.54 mg, 45% DRI
Vitamin B-6: 0.37 mg, 25% DRI
Zinc: 3.5 mg, 38% DRI

Health Benefits

Wheat germ has more nutrients per ounce than any other grain or vegetable. One 3.5 ounce serving of wheat germ provides 27 grams of protein, which is more protein per volume than most meats. Wheat germ is one of the richest sources of vitamin E and also provides a significant amount of omega-3 fatty acids. Here are some of the benefits of eating wheat germ.

- Wheat germ contains octacsanol, a substance that can lower cholesterol and improve muscle energy and endurance.
- A phytonutrient called beta-sitosterol, found in wheat germ, has been shown to inhibit the growth of prostate cancer cells.
- The high fiber content in wheat germ makes it helpful in maintaining regularity as well as preventing and treating constipation, diarrhea, diverticular disease, hemorrhoids, and irritable bowel syndrome.
- The high selenium in wheat germ may protect against cancer, because selenium activates glutathione peroxidase, a very potent antioxidant enzyme. Research shows that the lower the intake of selenium, the higher the incidence of cancer.
- B vitamins (e.g., thiamin, B-6, folate) benefit brain function and may help prevent and treat anxiety, depression, dementia, and memory loss.
- Selenium provides protection against heart attack and other cardiovascular conditions, according to recent research.

- Wheat germ is an excellent source of zinc, which may be helpful in the prevention and treatment of acne, colds, ear infections, infertility, prostate problems, and ulcers.

How to Select and Store

Because of its high oil content, keep wheat germ refrigerated and in a tightly sealed glass container. Even when refrigerated, wheat germ does not stay fresh for more than two to three months, so only buy as much as you plan to use within that time.

SWEET POTATO LATKES
Serves 6
2 cups shredded sweet potatoes
1 cup chopped onion
1 cup wheat germ
2 egg whites
½ tsp black pepper
Dash salt

Preheat oven to 400° F. Lightly grease two large cookie sheets. In a large bowl, combine all ingredients and mix well. Drop by ¼ cupfuls onto the cookie sheets and press with the bottom of a large glass to form 12 patties. Bake for 15 minutes, then turn and bake for 10–12 additional minutes until brown and crisp.

TOASTED WHEAT GERM
Makes ¼ cup
¼ cup wheat germ

Spread wheat germ on a baking sheet and bake for 5 minutes at 350° F. Use as a topping on yogurt, vegetable salads, fruit salad, soups, casseroles, cereal, and puddings, and in recipes for breads, muffins, cookies, cakes, pancakes, and rolls.

YOGURT

In recent years, yogurt has become the "in" food. This fermented dairy product, which is made by adding healthful strains of bacteria to milk, is being marketed in a growing number of flavors and varieties, with "special" yogurts targeted for children, women, and people with digestive conditions.

The word "yogurt" comes from the Turkish name *yoghurmak*, which means "to thicken." When the bacteria are added to milk—e.g., *Lactobacillus bulgaricus*, *L. acidophilus*, *Streptococcus thermophilus*—they transform the milk's sugar, lactose, into lactic acid. This process is what gives yogurt its puddinglike texture and tart flavor. Although it is unclear when yogurt was first developed, records of its use exist from the thirteenth century, when Genghis Khan's army ate it as a staple in their diet. Today yogurt is an important part of the diet in Turkey, India, the Middle East, Eastern Europe, and Asia.

Yogurt Nutrition
Serving Size: 1 cup, plain, low-fat
Calories: 154
Protein: 13 g
Total Fat: 3.8 g
Carbohydrates: 17 g
Fiber: 0 g
Cholesterol: 15 mg
Calcium: 448 mg, 45% DRI
Riboflavin: 0.5 mg, 41% DRI
Vitamin B-12: 1.4 mcg, 58% DRI

Health Benefits
Yogurt is an excellent source of calcium, but it is also a rich source of another type of healthful substance: probiotics, or beneficial bacteria. Together these ingredients make yogurt a wise choice for your health.

• In a study published in *Annals of Nutrition and Metabolism*, experts reported that women who ate yogurt daily had more than a thirty percent increase in the special white blood cells that fight infections, and that this boost to the immune system persisted even after the women stopped eating yogurt.

- Yogurt may help prevent vaginal yeast infections. Among women who had frequent yeast infections, those who ate eight ounces of yogurt daily for six months had a threefold decrease in infections.

- As little as three ounces of yogurt daily may reduce "bad" (LDL) cholesterol and raise "good" (HDL) cholesterol levels, according to a study in *Annals of Nutrition and Metabolism.*

- Yogurt is good for your bones. Along with calcium, yogurt also contains lactoferrin, a protein that boosts the activity and growth of osteoblasts—the cells that build bone—as well as decreases the formation of osteoclasts, which break down bone.

- Yogurt can effectively stop the activity of *Helicobacter pylori*, the bacterium that causes ulcers. A study in the *American Journal of Clinical Nutrition* found that daily consumption of yogurt effectively treated people who had ulcers caused by *H. pylori*.

- The probiotics in yogurt can reduce the formation of dental plaque and cavities, and the risk for gingivitis.

- The probiotics in yogurt also promote and maintain intestinal health; that is, they help prevent diarrhea, constipation, irritable bowel syndrome, colitis, diverticular disease, colorectal cancer, and other intestinal conditions, as well as maintain regularity.

How to Select and Store

Select organic yogurt and those that say "live active cultures" or "living yogurt cultures" on the label, and that contain at least two different strains of bacteria. Avoid yogurts that contain artificial flavors, sweeteners, or colors.

Store yogurt in the refrigerator. Unopened yogurt should stay fresh for about one week past the expiration date.

GREEN YOGURT SOUP
Serves 6
1 large zucchini
1 large cucumber
1¼ cup plain nonfat yogurt
⅓ cup nonfat milk
1 clove garlic
¼ tsp salt
Juice of one lemon

Chop the zucchini and cucumber into large chunks. Remove the seeds. Place all ingredients into a blender or food processor and blend until smooth. Chill for several hours. Add more milk before serving if the soup is too thick.

YOGURT-RICE SALAD
Serves 4
2 cups cooked brown rice
1½ cups nonfat plain yogurt
½ cup nonfat milk
1 cup chopped cucumber
¼ cup grated carrot
¼ cup chopped bell pepper
¼ cup chopped walnuts (optional)
Salt to taste
1 Tbs chopped cilantro leaves

Combine all ingredients in a bowl, mix well, and serve either at room temperature or chilled.

Top 20 Supplements

ALPHA-LIPOIC ACID

Alpha-lipoic acid (ALA) is a sulfur-containing fatty acid present in every cell in the human body. It is not a vitamin, because the body is capable of manufacturing it, yet scientists are not completely certain how ALA is produced. They do know that its main function is to generate energy, which it does in many energy-producing processes. It also is a potent antioxidant that has the special ability to function in both water-soluble and fat-soluble environments, which means it can enhance the activities of both types of vitamins (e.g., water-soluble ones like vitamin C and fat-soluble, like vitamin E). Without lipoic acid, these two antioxidants could not survive in the body.

Health Benefits

The human body cannot maximize energy production from fats and carbohydrates without ALA. Alpha-lipoic acid also has a hand in many other processes in the body.

- Many studies show that ALA can improve symptoms associated with diabetes, including neuropathy and retinopathy.
- Numerous studies also show that ALA improves insulin sensitivity and glucose metabolism in people who have type 2 diabetes.
- Lipoic acid appears to be helpful in the prevention and treatment of age-related memory loss and dementia.
- Some research suggests ALA can help in weight loss by reducing the desire to eat and slightly increasing metabolism.
- Taking ALA supplements may help reduce the risk of heart disease, stroke, and cataracts because this nutrient inhibits lipid peroxidation—a process in which free radicals damage fat cells.
- Alpha-lipoic acid may offer some protection against nerve cell damage associated with stroke.

How Much Do I Need?

No daily requirement has been established for ALA. Many health-care practitioners recommend 25–50 mg per day to maintain health, but higher doses may be suggested for specific conditions, such as memory loss. Dosages greater than 100 mg daily may cause nausea and abnormally low blood sugar.

Interactions

No negative interactions with drugs have been noted. Alpha-lipoic acid interacts positively with the antioxidant vitamins C and E, coenzyme Q, and glutathione, all of which need ALA to function efficiently. If you have a deficiency of sulfur-containing amino acids (e.g., cysteine, taurine, methionine), your body will be unable to synthesize a sufficient amount of ALA.

Food Sources

Only a few foods contain ALA, including broccoli, greens, liver, and yeast.

BIOFLAVONOIDS

The bioflavonoids are a group of more than 5,000 plant pigments, many of which are known for their antioxidant powers. We look at them collectively rather than individually because they share this free-radical-fighting ability, many of them are combined and made available in supplement form, and because we don't have the space to discuss each one! (Exceptions are lycopene, lutein, and zeaxanthin, which are covered separately in this chapter.) Experts are continually discovering more ways bioflavonoids are important to health and well-being. Some of the more commonly recognized and studied bioflavonoids include anthocyanins, catechins, flavonols, isoflavones, quercetin, proanthocyanidins, reservatrol, and rutin.

Health Benefits

Let's look at a few of these bioflavonoids and their benefits.

- Quercetin inhibits the release of histamine, which makes it helpful in the treatment of allergies and inflammation.
- A high intake of quercetin may reduce your risk of type 2 diabetes and lower the mortality rate from ischemic heart disease.

- Quercetin has proven useful in the treatment of prostatitis.
- Pycnogenol®, an extract from French maritime pine bark, boosts the immune system and helps prevent and treat varicose veins. Animal studies indicate that it may also help treat inflammatory bowel disease.
- Rutin and hesperidin work with vitamin C to maintain healthy capillaries, form collagen in connective tissue (and thus is beneficial for arthritis), and support a healthy immune system.
- Hesperidin is helpful in treating hemorrhoids and varicose veins.
- Researchers note that a high intake of flavonoids is associated with a very low incidence of asthma.
- Proanthocyanidins found in cranberries are effective in preventing urinary tract infections.
- Growing evidence shows that the flavonoids found in berries (blueberries, cranberries, etc.) can limit the development and severity of certain cancers and vascular diseases such as atherosclerosis and stroke.

How Much Do I Need?

No minimum daily requirement has been established for bioflavonoids, but generally 500 mg per day is suggested. Bioflavonoids should be taken along with vitamin C, and many supplements conveniently contain both.

Interactions

A few interactions between bioflavonoid supplements and medications have been noted.

- The citrus flavonoid tangeretin interferes with the ability of tamoxifen to prohibit tumor growth. If you are taking tamoxifen, it is probably best to avoid taking any citrus bioflavonoid supplements.
- Use of flavonoid supplements could reduce the effectiveness of many anticancer drugs and radiation

treatments. Such supplements can be used once treatment has stopped.

- The bioflavonoid naringin increases the effect of calcium channel blockers, drugs such as nifedipine, verapamil, and felodipine. Naringin also inhibits the breakdown of estrogens and coumarin, and should not be used when taking any of these medications.

Food Sources

Bioflavonoids are found in many foods, some of which include apples, apricots, buckwheat, bell peppers, blueberries, broccoli, cherries, citrus (grapefruit, lemons, oranges; in the white material just beneath the peel are the richest sources), cranberries, garlic, grapes, green tea, and onions.

CALCIUM

Say "calcium" and most people think "bones," and that's a good place to begin. Of the approximately one thousand grams of calcium found in the average adult, nearly ninety-eight percent of it is in bone, one percent is in teeth, and the remaining amount is in the blood, other bodily fluids, and within cells. Calcium is the most abundant mineral in the human body, and it is responsible for many critical processes, including blood clotting, muscle tone, nerve conduction, muscle contractions, and heart health.

Health Benefits

Let's put bone health aside for a moment and consider the minute but critically important amount of calcium in your blood. This calcium is needed for life-giving processes, so if you do not get an adequate amount daily, your body takes the calcium that it needs from your bones and puts it into your bloodstream. Over time, your bones will lose an increasing amount of calcium and place you at high risk of developing osteoporosis. Some of the residual calcium that leaves the bones can get into joints and cause arthritis, or bind with fat and form plaque in the arteries. Therefore, getting enough calcium is about more than bone health!

- Calcium and vitamin D can reduce symptoms of PMS.
- Several studies show that calcium can help reduce the risk of colon cancer, as calcium binds with bile and fatty acids in the colon, substances which are known to stimulate cancer cell production.
- Supplementation with calcium has been shown to reduce high blood pressure.
- The risk of colon cancer appears to be reduced in people who take calcium supplements. One large study found that adults who took 700–800 mg of calcium daily had a 40–50 percent reduced risk of developing colon cancer.
- Several studies indicate that higher intake of calcium is associated with lower body weight or less tendency to gain weight over time.

How Much Do I Need?

The DRI for calcium for both men and women is 1,000–1,200 mg daily. When buying supplements, look for the amount of elemental calcium in each dose, which is the amount of calcium the body can absorb. To determine the amount of elemental calcium, look at the Percent Daily Value (%DV) on the label. The %DV is based on 1,000 mg of elemental calcium, so every ten percent in the DV column represents 100 mg of elemental calcium. For example, if a calcium supplement has 50%DV, it contains 500 mg of elemental calcium. Choose either calcium citrate (best absorbed and available in liquid) or calcium carbonate (most common form).

Interactions

Calcium supplements can interact with various drugs and supplements. Here are the highlights.

- Corticosteroids (e.g., prednisone, hydrocortisone) reduce the body's ability to activate vitamin D, which leads to a decrease in calcium absorption and increased excretion of calcium in urine.

- Some antibiotics (e.g., gentamicin, erythromycin, neomycin, tobramycin) may hinder calcium absorption or use by the body.
- Hormone replacement therapy may decrease calcium excretion and increase calcium absorption in post-menopausal women.
- Anticonvulsant medications (e.g., Dilantin) may result in reduced calcium absorption.
- Calcium supplements may interfere with the absorption of alendronate (Fosamax®), which is used to treat and prevent osteoporosis.
- High intake of sodium, caffeine, or protein causes an increase in the amount of calcium excreted in urine.
- Calcium in both food and supplements can reduce the amount of iron the body absorbs.
- Because calcium and magnesium compete for absorption in the intestinal tract, take these supplements about two hours apart.

Food Sources

Calcium in food is absorbed better than that in supplements. You can boost the amount of calcium your body absorbs from food and supplements if you eat vitamin C–rich food when you consume calcium. Foods that supply a good amount of calcium include almonds, beans, broccoli, cheese (low-fat), greens, nonfat milk, salmon (with bones), soy (calcium-fortified), tofu, and yogurt.

COENZYME Q10

Coenzyme Q10 (CoQ10), or ubiquinone, is a fat-soluble, vitamin-like substance that is found in very small amounts in many foods and is also synthesized in all tissues from the amino acid tyrosine. CoQ10 is a potent antioxidant and is necessary for basic cell functioning. Levels of CoQ10 decline with age and often are also low in people who have chronic diseases such as cancer, diabetes, heart disease, Parkinson's disease, and HIV/AIDS.

Health Benefits

Experts are investigating the potential benefits of CoQ10, but the results are preliminary in many cases. Here are some of the advantages researchers have found thus far.

- Dozens of clinical studies show that CoQ10 significantly improves heart function, and therefore appears to be helpful in preventing and treating atherosclerosis, heart attack, stroke, and other cardiovascular conditions.
- So far, several animals studies have shown that CoQ10 boosts the immune system, helps fight infections, and may help stop cancer cells from growing.
- Several studies show that taking 150 mg or 300 mg of CoQ10 daily reduced the frequency of migraine attacks.

How Much Do I Need?

Experts have not established a DRI for CoQ10. The average therapeutic dose is 100 to 300 mg daily, although it can go higher depending on the condition you are treating. Side effects are typically mild and brief, and may include nausea, vomiting, heartburn, diarrhea, rash, headache, and low blood sugar.

Interactions

Generally, CoQ10 can be used safely along with medications and other supplements. If you are using any of the following products, however, an interaction may occur.

- Drugs used to reduce cholesterol or blood sugar levels may reduce the effects of CoQ10.
- Statin drugs (e.g., lovastatin, pravastatin, simvastatin), which treat high blood pressure, can significantly reduce the body's ability to synthesize CoQ10.

- Use of CoQ10 may alter the way your body uses warfarin and insulin.

Food Sources

The highest levels of CoQ10 are found in red meat, especially organ meat, but it is also available in beans (dried), carrots, cauliflower, eggs, garlic, olive oil, peanuts, soy, sweet potatoes, walnuts, and yogurt.

FIBER

You grandmother may have called it roughage or bulk, but today we refer to it as "dietary fiber," the parts of plant foods that your body cannot absorb or digest. Fiber has gotten a bad rap, but you would be miserable without it. Not only does fiber help keep you "regular," but it offers many other health benefits as well.

Fiber is either soluble (dissolves in water and forms a gel-like substance) or insoluble (does not dissolve in water). Plant foods contain both types, although the amount present in each food varies. The two types of fiber provide different benefits, so it is best to eat a variety of high-fiber foods so you can enjoy the advantages of both.

Health Benefits

The best way to remember the main benefits of the two types of fiber is this: *in*soluble fiber works *in*side the *in*testinal tract to *in*crease the transport of material through the digestive system, while soluble fiber reduces glucose and cholesterol levels. Here are some specifics:

- Insoluble fiber increases stool bulk and consistency, which in turn helps prevent constipation and, if loose stools are a problem, can help add bulk and eliminate diarrhea.
- A high-fiber diet may reduce your risk of hemorrhoids, colon cancer, diverticulitis, and irritable bowel syndrome.

- Research shows that soluble fiber can lower blood cholesterol levels and slow the absorption of glucose (sugar), which can improve blood sugar levels for people with diabetes.
- A high-fiber diet can help fight obesity. When you eat high-fiber foods, you feel full and stay satisfied longer. High-fiber foods also tend to have fewer calories, which means you may eat more food but consume fewer calories.

How Much Do I Need?

The Institutes of Medicine recommend that adults fifty years and younger consume twenty-one grams (women) and thirty grams (men) per day; after age fifty, women need twenty-five grams and men thirty-eight grams. Most adults to not reach these goals, because processed foods, which are a staple of the American diet, lack sufficient fiber.

The best way to meet your daily fiber requirement is to eat more fresh fruits and vegetables, beans, and whole-grain foods, as they provide important nutrients along with the fiber. If you need additional fiber, look for fiber supplements that contain natural ingredients, such as psyllium husks or methylcellulose.

Interactions

Fiber supplements can interfere with various medications.

- Absorption of anti-diabetic medications, especially glyburide and metforming, may be reduced if taken at the same time as fiber supplements.
- The body's ability to absorb digoxin may be reduced if taken along with fiber supplements. Take fiber two hours before or after your medication.
- If you are taking lithium, psyllium or other soluble fiber may reduce the effectiveness of this drug.
- On a positive note, use of psyllium or other soluble fibers along with colestipol or cholestyramine can enhance the ability of your body to reduce cholesterol levels.

Food Sources

Fruits, vegetables, grains, legumes, and seeds typically contain both types of fiber, and although the balance is sometimes in favor of one or the other, it is best to eat a variety of high-fiber foods rather than worry about which "type" of fiber you are getting. Better sources of fiber include apples, barley, beans (dried, cooked), broccoli, brown rice, carrots, flaxseed, lentils, oats, oranges, pears, peas, squash, whole grains, and 100% bran cereals.

FOLIC ACID

Folic acid, also referred to as vitamin B-9, belongs to the B family of vitamins. The natural form of this vitamin that occurs in food is folate; the synthetic form used in supplements and added to foods is folic acid. Regardless of the form, vitamin B-9 helps produce and maintain new cells, DNA, and RNA, and helps prevent changes to DNA that may result in cancer.

Health Benefits

Folate plays many critical roles, but perhaps it is best known for helping to prevent birth defects. In fact, in 1996 the Food and Drug Administration (FDA) required food manufacturers to fortify grain products with folic acid to help ensure women would get a sufficient amount of the vitamin. Other benefits of folate are discussed here.

- Folic acid supplementation can reduce homocysteine levels, which may in turn reduce your risk of heart disease and stroke.
- High intake of folate has been linked with a reduced risk of breast cancer in postmenopausal women.
- A 2007 meta-analysis of eight trials found that folic acid supplements reduced the risk of stroke by eighteen percent.
- Folic acid can relieve the symptoms of psoriasis.

- Some studies suggest that folic acid supplementation may help fight depression and/or enhance the effectiveness of medications taken to treat depression. Research shows a forty-two percent greater risk of depression in people with low levels of folate.

How Much Do I Need?

The DRI for folic acid is 400 mcg for adults. If you are pregnant, the recommended dose is 800 mcg daily. The suggested dose for people who have elevated homocysteine levels is 1,000–2,000 mcg daily. Side effects are rare, and may include sleep disruptions and intestinal discomfort.

Interactions

Be aware of the following interactions that may occur if you are taking any of the following drugs while supplementing with folic acid.

- The following medications can deplete folic acid from the body: aspirin and other nonsteroidal antiinflammatory drugs, barbiturates, choline magnesium, corticosteroids, oral contraceptives, primidone, and ranitidine.
- Methotrexate can impair the conversion of folic acid in the body and result in low levels or deficiency. If you are taking methotrexate to treat arthritis or psoriasis, 1,000 mcg of folic acid should be taken to prevent deficiency. If, however, you are taking methotrexate for cancer, a folic acid supplement can reduce the effectiveness of the drug and should not be used during treatment.
- Use of proton pump inhibitors (e.g., esomoprazole, lansoprazole, omeprazole) may reduce your body's ability to absorb folic acid; therefore, folic acid supplementation may be necessary while using these drugs.
- Simultaneous use of phenytoin (antiseizure medication) and folic acid (1,000 mcg or greater per day) may

reduce the effectiveness of the drug and cause an increase in seizures.
- Use of folic acid supplements along with vitamin B-12
supplements may increase the risk of a B-12 deficiency.

Food Sources

Sources of folate include avocados, bananas, beans (dried),
broccoli, cantaloupe, eggs, lettuce, papaya, peas, spinach, and
wheat germ.

INDOLE-3-CARBINOL

Indole-3-carbinol is a phytonutrient found in cruciferous vegetables, such as broccoli, cabbage, and cauliflower. This naturally occurring nutrient is made from indole-3-glucosinolate
when it is activated by a special enzyme that springs into action when the vegetables are chewed.

Health Benefits

Indole-3-carbinol is mainly known as a potent antioxidant
that helps prevent free-radical damage to the body's cells, and
as an anticancer nutrient.

- Numerous studies show indole-3-carbinol can help
  prevent estrogen-dependent cancers, including breast,
  cervical, ovarian, and endometrial cancers, because it
  blocks estrogen receptor sites on the membranes of
  breast and other cells.
- This phytonutrient has anticlotting abilities, which may
  make it helpful in preventing stroke and heart attack.
- A few studies suggest indole-3-carbinol may help prevent prostate cancer, but much more research is
  needed in this area.

How Much Do I Need?

No daily requirement has been established for indole-3-
carbinol. Dose levels used in cancer-prevention studies gener-

ally range from 200 to 400 mg daily. No side effects have been reported.

Interactions

Supplements of indole-3-carbinol may affect how your body metabolizes the following drugs. Talk to your doctor before taking indole-3-carbinol with: clozapine, cyclobenzaprine, fluvoxamine, haloperidol, imipramine, mexiletine, nicotine, olanzapine, pentazocine, propranolol, tacrine, tamoxifen, theophylline, and zolmitriptan.

Food Sources

The cruciferous vegetables are the main sources of indole-3-carbinol. They include broccoli, brussels sprouts, cabbage, cauliflower, greens, radishes, and turnips.

LUTEIN AND ZEAXANTHIN

Lutein and zeaxanthin are two important carotenoids that are abundant in many fruits, vegetables, and some whole grains. We look at these two potent antioxidants together for three reasons: statistical information on them is typically reported together; they are usually found together in the same foods; and they are most often associated with the eyes, where they are both found in very high concentrations in the retina.

Most Americans do not consume enough foods that are rich in lutein; in fact, the majority of people get only 1–2 mg daily instead of the 6 mg or more suggested. Supplements can help fill in the gap, but it's still best to get most of your lutein and zeaxanthin by eating more fruits and vegetables.

Health Benefits

The antioxidant capabilities of both lutein and zeaxanthin offer several important benefits. Here's a rundown of the research.

- In the fight against atherosclerosis, lutein appears to be helpful in reducing buildup of plaque in the walls of arteries.
- Studies show that people who get the most lutein and zeaxanthin in their diets are protected against cataracts and macular degeneration.
- Several studies suggest lutein and zeaxanthin, along with other carotenoids, may protect against development of breast cancer.

How Much Do I Need?

No Daily Values have been established for lutein and zeaxanthin, but research suggests a minimum of 6–10 mg of lutein daily is needed to reap its benefits. Lutein/zeaxanthin supplements are most often made from marigolds, a rich source of both phytonutrients. The ratio of lutein to zeaxanthin in marigolds is typically around 20:1, so if the supplement label says a dose contains 4 mg of lutein, you will also be getting 0.2 mg of zeaxanthin.

Supplements differ greatly, so read labels carefully. Lutein and zeaxanthin are often part of combination supplements that also contain other antioxidants, such as vitamin A/beta-carotene, vitamin C, vitamin E, and/or zinc and copper, all of which are important for eye health. No side effects have been reported.

Interactions

No interactions with drugs, foods, or other supplements have been noted.

Food Sources

Lutein is found in many vegetables, including butternut squash, corn, cucumbers, green bell peppers, kale, kiwi, pumpkin, red grapes, spinach, and zucchini squash. Zeaxanthin is abundant in orange bell peppers (an excellent source), corn, spinach, collards, oranges, mango, and tangerines, and in good levels in green beans, peas, broccoli, celery, and peaches.

LYCOPENE

Lycopene is a member of the carotenoid family of phytonutrients, and is the pigment that gives tomatoes and several other fruits and vegetables their color. More than eighty percent of the lycopene consumed in the United States is in the form of tomato sauce, pizza, and ketchup, and it is the number one carotenoid eaten in the United States (beta-carotene is number two). Experts became interested in lycopene in the late 1980s when they discovered that it had twice the antioxidant power of beta-carotene and that it appeared to help fight against some cancers.

Health Benefits

Studies show that people who eat cooked tomatoes have higher levels of lycopene in their blood than those who eat raw tomatoes or drink tomato juice. Thus lycopene is better used by the body when the tomatoes are cooked. Whether you eat lots of cooked tomatoes and tomato products and/or take lycopene supplements, here are some of lycopene's health benefits.

- Asthma sufferers can enjoy some protection from symptoms if they take lycopene and/or eat lycopene-rich foods, according to recent research.
- The risk of prostate cancer appears to be reduced in men who consume lycopene.
- Lycopene may help reduce the risk of colon cancer, as well as other types of cancer, according to recent studies.
- Research indicates that a combination of lycopene and green tea offers potent protection against prostate cancer.
- Eating foods rich in lycopene can inhibit the damage caused by LDL cholesterol and in turn reduce the risk of heart disease.
- Laboratory studies indicate that lycopene may help prevent age-related macular degeneration.

• Some studies show that lycopene is helpful in treating infertility in men, but additional research is needed.

How Much Do I Need?

Lycopene supplements are available in softgels and capsules, and are usually sold in a combination form, along with lutein, beta-carotene, and other carotenoids. No specific doses have been established for lycopene; however, based on scientific studies, the following amounts have been beneficial: 30 mg daily for adults with exercise-induced asthma; 1.2 g of 6% lycopene oleoresin for adults with atherosclerosis; and at least 6.5 mg for men with prostate cancer. Consult your doctor before taking lycopene supplements.

No side effects associated with lycopene supplements have been noted.

Interactions

The interaction of lycopene supplements with drugs or supplements has not been well researched. However, here is what some experts say.

• In theory, lycopene may increase the cholesterol-lowering effects of lovastatin or other statin drugs, or use of these drugs may decrease the amount of lycopene in the blood. Other drugs that may reduce the amount of lycopene in the body include cholestyramine, colestipol, nicotine, and alcohol.
• Some positive interactions also occur. For example, inhibition of the growth of cancerlike cells increases when lycopene is used with vitamins D or E, and its antioxidant effects are increased when it is used along with lutein.

Food Sources

Along with tomatoes and tomato products (e.g., ketchup, tomato paste, tomato juice), lycopene is found in significant amounts in apricots, guava, pink grapefruit, watermelon, and papaya.

MAGNESIUM

Magnesium is the fourth most abundant mineral in the body and a nutrient that often gets mentioned along with calcium, as a balance of these two minerals is essential for healthy bones and normal muscle function (see below). Indeed, about sixty-five percent of the body's magnesium is in the bones and teeth. However, magnesium also plays a critical role in more than three hundred enzymatic reactions in the body.

Health Benefits

- Magnesium and calcium work together to maintain normal muscle function: calcium makes muscles contract, while magnesium is necessary to help them relax and prevent restriction of blood vessels that can occur when muscles contract.
- Studies suggest that magnesium may reduce the risk of stroke and coronary heart disease. There is also evidence that low magnesium levels may increase the risk of abnormal heart rhythms.
- Magnesium helps maintain normal blood pressure. A four-year study of more than thirty thousand male health professionals found that a lower risk of hypertension was associated with a diet that contained more magnesium, potassium, and fiber.
- Common infections like colds, flu, bronchitis, and sinusitis are better prevented when the immune system is supported by adequate levels of magnesium.
- Magnesium may help regulate blood sugar levels and thus benefit people who have diabetes, especially those who have low blood levels of the mineral (hypomagnesemia), a frequent occurrence among individuals with type 2 diabetes.
- Magnesium is necessary for protein synthesis and energy metabolism.

How Much Do I Need?

The Institute of Medicine has established the DRI for magnesium for adults as 310 mg (females) and 420 mg (males). Talk to your doctor before taking magnesium supplements if you have kidney disease. Taking more than 750 mg of magnesium daily can cause diarrhea and drowsiness. As a supplement, magnesium glycinate is recommended because it is well absorbed and is less likely to cause loose stools, which is a side effect of this mineral.

Low levels of magnesium can cause or contribute to kidney stones, arrhythmia, tachycardia, coronary artery spasm, premenstrual syndrome, menstrual cramps, high blood pressure, mitral valve prolapse, tetany (sustained convulsions or contractions), chronic constipation, insomnia, and hyperactivity (especially in children).

Interactions

Use of magnesium supplements while taking any of the following medications can lead to undesirable interactions.

- Loop and thiazide diuretics, antibiotics, and antineoplastic drugs may increase the loss of magnesium in urine, resulting in a magnesium deficiency.
- Magnesium binds to tetracycline, which reduces the body's ability to absorb the medication.

Food Sources

Rich sources of magnesium include almonds, avocados, brown rice, bananas, greens, lentils, oats, soybeans, and tofu.

OMEGA-3 FATTY ACIDS

Essential omega-3 fatty acids are thus named because they are needed to maintain good health, but the body cannot manufacture them. Therefore it is "essential" that you get omega-3s from your diet, as well as supplementation as needed. The three major types of omega-3 fatty acids in food are alpha-linolenic acid (ALA), eicosapentaenoic acid (EPA), and do-cosahexaenoic acid (DHA). When you eat foods that contain ALA, the body converts it to EPA and DHA, forms that are more easily used by the body.

Omega-3s are part of the polyunsaturated fat family, which is also occupied by omega-6, another essential fatty acid (EFA). An appropriate balance between these two EFAs is important to help maintain and improve health. The desirable balance is about 4:1 of omega-6 to omega-3, yet most Americans have a ratio of 25:1 or greater, which many experts believe is a major reason behind the growing number of inflammatory problems in the United States, including heart disease and arthritis.

Health Benefits

Many of the health benefits associated with omega-3s are related to their ability to reduce inflammation (while most omega-6 EFAs promote it), but omega-3s offer other advantages as well. Here's a rundown.

- Studies show that walnuts (which are rich in ALA) and fish oil supplements that contain EPA and DHA reduce bad cholesterol (low-density lipoprotein, LDL) and triglyceride levels in people who have high levels of these unhealthy substances.
- Omega-3 EFA supplements (3 g daily) can reduce high blood pressure, thus lowering your risk of heart disease and stroke.
- Consuming omega-3 EFAs reduces the risk of stroke by preventing the buildup of plaque and the formation of blood clots in the arteries that lead to the brain.
- Omega-3 EFA supplements reduce joint tenderness, morning stiffness, and the need for medication among people who have rheumatoid arthritis.
- Improvements in grip strength, pain, joint stiffness, and walking pace have been seen in people who take omega-3 EFAs.
- Omega-3 EFAs benefit women who suffer with painful menstruation associated with PMS.

- Improved bone strength and increased calcium levels in bone have been attributed to omega-3 EFAs, which in turn reduces women's risk of developing osteoporosis.
- Omega-3 EFAs assist in nerve cell communication, which is key in maintaining mood. A healthy ratio of omega-6 to omega-3 is also needed to avoid depression.
- Studies show that the addition of omega-3 EFAs to medication for inflammatory bowel diseases (e.g., ulcerative colitis, Crohn's disease) can reduce symptoms.
- Adult asthma sufferers may experience reduced inflammation and an improvement in lung function when taking omega-3 EFA supplements.
- Omega-3 EFAs may protect against prostate, breast, and colon cancers. Because there is some question about ALA causing an increased risk of prostate cancer, it is best to take supplements that contain EPA and DHA rather than ALA.
- Omega-3s are especially important for sperm production and motility, as DHA is found in high concentrations in sperm.

How Much Do I Need?

For healthy adults, the Adequate Intake established by the Institute of Medicine for ALA is 1.1 to 1.6 g per day, but it has not established values for EPA and DHA. The World Health Organization (WHO) and other world government organizations recommend 0.3 to 0.5 g of EPA plus DHA daily, along with 0.8 to 1.1 g of ALA daily. Flaxseed oil supplements provide ALA, fish-oil supplements provide EPA and DHA, and those made from algae provide DHA.

Side effects of omega-3 supplements may include fishy aftertaste (if using fish oil), gas, flatulence, and nausea.

Interactions

Omega-3 supplements can interact with certain medications, so check with your doctor if you take any of the following drugs.

- Omega-3 supplements may alter the effects of blood-thinning drugs (e.g., aspirin, warfarin) by increasing the risk of bleeding and bruising.
- Drugs that lower blood sugar (e.g., glipizide, glyburide, insulin) may not be as effective if you take omega-3 EFAs.
- If you have high cholesterol and are taking cholesterol-reducing drugs (e.g., statins), including omega-3s in your diet may help these drugs to work more effectively.
- If you are taking cyclosporine, taking omega-3s may reduce the drug's toxic side effects.

Food Sources

The richest sources of EPA and DHA are cold-water fish such as halibut, herring, mackerel, salmon, sardines, and tuna, while ALA is found in canola oil, flaxseed, pumpkin seeds, purslane, soybeans, and walnuts.

PROBIOTICS

Probiotics are live microorganisms that are similar to those that live in the digestive and intestinal tract in the body. As a supplement they are unique because they are composed of bacteria, which most people consider to be harmful, but in this case, they are beneficial (friendly). Probiotics can both maintain health and treat various medical conditions.

Probiotics usually belong to one of two groups: *Bifidobacterium* or *Lactobacillus*. Each group (genus) has different species (e.g., *L. acidophilus* and *B. bifidus*) and strains. Foods that contain beneficial bacteria have been used for millennia, such as yogurt and fermented dairy products, and their health benefits have long been recognized. Yet it is only recently that experts have begun to understand the science behind those benefits.

Health Benefits

Probiotics can be helpful in both preventing and treating a wide variety of ailments.

- Probiotics can prevent or treat symptoms associated with the use of antibiotics—diarrhea, gas, bloating, high risk of developing yeast infections. It is best to begin taking probiotics (and/or eating foods that contain probiotics) as soon as you know you will be taking an antibiotic. Continue to take the probiotics throughout the antibiotic treatment and for one to two weeks after completing your medication.
- Probiotics have been shown to eliminate or significantly reduce symptoms of infectious diarrhea, irritable bowel syndrome, Crohn's disease, inflammatory bowel disease, and other gastrointestinal problems.
- Several studies show probiotics can significantly reduce the risk of eczema in infants.
- The probiotics *Lactobacillus reuteri* can reduce the risk of developing gingivitis and its symptoms, such as gum bleeding and plaque buildup.
- Women with urinary tract infections may get relief or prevent recurrent infection if they take probiotics.
- Some probiotics (various *Lactobacillus* species) have been effective against vaginitis, including yeast infections caused by Candida.

How Much Do I Need?

No daily requirement has been established for beneficial bacteria. Some experts recommend taking one to two billion CFUs (colony-forming units, the standard by which probiotics are measured) daily of at least four different species (available in a combination supplement) as a preventive measure and to maintain health. Higher doses are usually suggested when treating a specific condition; generally, ten to fifteen CFUs per day until the symptoms clear.

Interactions

The only interaction associated with probiotics is an increased need for these beneficial bacteria if you are taking antibiotics. Use of antibiotics destroys both bad and good bacteria, which then places you at risk for developing many symptoms or conditions, including diarrhea, urinary tract infections, yeast infections, and digestive disorders.

Food Sources

Foods that contain beneficial bacteria include fermented vegetables, kefir, tempeh, yogurt, and an increasing number of foods that are fortified with probiotics, including some cereals, cottage cheese, and nutrition bars. Always read the label to determine which probiotics are in the product and the amount.

SELENIUM

Selenium is a mineral that was not recognized for its essential role in human health until the 1960s. Today it is valued as an antioxidant, and works with vitamin E and as part of a critically important enzyme called glutathione peroxidase, which is a potent free-radical fighter.

Health Benefits

Generally, selenium protects red blood cells from free-radical damage, boosts the immune system, helps produce prostaglandins (substances that affect inflammation and blood pressure), and fights the effects of toxic minerals in the body. Here are some more specific benefits offered by this mineral.

- Taking supplemental selenium can help boost your immune system and make it more resistant against the common cold, flu, bronchitis, sinusitis, and other viral and bacterial infections.
- Selenium supplementation can help asthmatics by reducing lung inflammation.

- Several studies indicate selenium may reduce the risk of some types of cancer, including lung and liver cancer, while the research on prostate cancer has yielded mixed results.
- In several studies, people with HIV who took 200 mcg of selenium daily for up to two years experienced an improvement in symptoms, CD4 T-cell counts, and progression of the virus.
- Supplementation with selenium has improved sperm motility in infertile men.

How Much Do I Need?

The DRI for selenium is 55 mcg for adults, and the suggested supplement dose is usually 100 to 200 mcg. Taking 1,000 mcg or more per day can cause adverse effects, including vomiting, diarrhea, fatigue, numbness, and loss of control in the legs and arms.

Interactions

Selenium is generally very safe, and interacts well with most other supplements and medications. There are some exceptions, however.

- Use of valproic acid (an anticonvulsant drug) can decrease plasma levels of selenium.
- Selenium may reduce the toxic side effects associated with two chemotherapy drugs, doxorubicin and cisplatin.
- Selenium may inhibit the anticancer effects of the chemotherapy drug bleomycin.

Food Sources

The amount of selenium in foods can vary significantly, as it depends on the amount of selenium in the soil in which the plants were grown and/or the foods consumed by the animals that are eaten. Generally, selenium levels are higher in organ meats and fish (e.g., salmon) than in plants, but there are many good plant sources as well, including Brazil nuts, brown rice, nonfat milk, and walnuts (black). Organic produce is much more likely to contain good levels of selenium.

VITAMIN A/BETA-CAROTENE

Why do we talk about these two nutrients together? Because beta-carotene is a precursor (something that precedes) of vitamin A; that is, when you consume the carotenoid beta-carotene, either in food or as a supplement, your body transforms it into vitamin A as it is needed. Thus you can get vitamin A in two ways: directly through animal-based foods in a form called retinol, or from plant-based foods, known as carotenoids.

There are advantages to obtaining your vitamin A from beta-carotene rather than retinol. Vitamin A is fat soluble, which means the body stores it. Excessive amounts of vitamin A can cause headache, joint and bone pain, liver damage, nerve damage, and other side effects. Although beta-carotene is also fat soluble, it does not cause these side effects: it is both safe and beneficial to the body at high doses, and has heart-protective and cancer-prevention features that vitamin A does not have. Thus, beta-carotene is the preferred way to get your vitamin A.

Health Benefits

Vitamin A/beta-carotene plays many crucial roles in the body.

- The immune system receives a great deal of support from the antioxidant powers of vitamin A/beta-carotene, which help it fight infections like bronchitis, the common cold, ear infections, gingivitis, sinusitis, and urinary tract infections.
- Your chances of having a stroke are greatly reduced and your chances of recovering from one are improved if your levels of vitamin A/beta-carotene are high.
- Beta-carotene promotes cell-to-cell communication, which appears to be essential in the prevention of cancer.

- Beta-carotene may also be helpful in the treatment of acne, cataracts, eczema, herpes, and psoriasis.

How Much Do I Need?

The DRI for vitamin A is 2,300 IU for women and 3,000 IU for men. When choosing a supplement, look for ones that provide vitamin A as beta-carotene, either alone or as part of a multiple-vitamin supplement. Although no DRI has been established for beta-carotene, the National Academy of Sciences and other health agencies urge people to eat five or more servings of fruits and vegetables daily, which should provide approximately three to six mg of beta-carotene daily.

Interactions

Beta-carotene supplements may interact with some medications and other nutrients.

- The cholesterol-reducing medications cholestyramine, colestipol, and colestid can lower blood levels of beta-carotene.
- Beta-carotene supplements may reduce levels of lutein in the blood.
- If you are taking pectin supplements, they may reduce your body's ability to absorb beta-carotene.

Food Sources

Vitamin A is found in animal-based foods, including butter, nonfat milk, and liver. Beta-carotene is abundant in plants, with some of the richest sources being apricots, cantaloupe, carrots, greens, oranges, pumpkin, tangerines, sweet potatoes, and yellow squash.

VITAMIN B-6 (PYRIDOXINE)

This member of the B-complex family of vitamins is much in demand; in fact, it is believed to support more bodily functions than any of the vitamins. More than a hundred enzymes involved in protein metabolism depend on vitamin B-6. Without vitamin B-6, red blood cell metabolism would not function properly, nor would the immune and nervous systems.

Health Benefits

Severe deficiencies of vitamin B-6 are rare, but mild deficiencies are common and can occur in people who have cirrhosis, poor diet, hyperthyroidism, congestive heart failure, malabsorption syndrome, or who abuse alcohol.

- Vitamin B-6 is necessary for the production of norepinephrine and serotonin, two chemicals involved with mood. Although researchers have not identified whether vitamin B-6 supplementation can improve mood, some experts recommend taking 25 to 100 mg daily to prevent depression.
- Taking vitamin B-6 supplements can lower levels of homocysteine, a goal worth achieving, as high levels of this substance are a risk factor for heart disease and stroke, and possibly for Alzheimer's disease and osteoporosis.
- The combination of folate and vitamin B-6 can help reduce the risk of heart attack.
- Supplementation with vitamin B-6 can relieve symptoms of PMS.
- Vitamin B-6 is critical for the manufacture of substances called prostaglandins, which are involved in blood pressure regulation, heart function, and platelet aggregation (clotting).
- Because vitamin B-6 is important in skin health, maintaining adequate levels may help in treating acne, eczema, psoriasis, and other skin disorders.

How Much Do I Need?

The DRI for vitamin B-6 is 1.3 to 1.7 mg for males and 1.3 to 1.5 mg for females. Food processing destroys much of the vitamin, so it is best to get vitamin B-6 from whole and fresh food sources. The suggested supplement dose is 25 to 100 mg daily; the liquid form is the best absorbed.

Interactions

If you take a vitamin B-6 supplement, you may not get its full benefits if you are also using any of the following drugs:

- Alcohol and tobacco reduce the absorption of vitamin B-6.
- Vitamin B-6 may prevent levodopa from controlling Parkinson's symptoms.
- Estrogen and oral contraceptives can reduce vitamin absorption rates.
- Isonicotinic acid hydrazide, isoniazid, hydralazine, penicillamine, and immunosuppressants increase the excretion of vitamin B-6 and can cause anemia.

Food Sources

Food sources of vitamin B-6 include avocado, banana, carrots, eggs, greens, lentils, oatmeal, peas, salmon, sweet potato, tuna, turkey, wheat germ, and whole grains.

VITAMIN B-12

Vitamin B-12 is an essential water-soluble vitamin that is found primarily in animal foods. Although it is water soluble, the body can store several years' worth of the vitamin, so nutritional deficiency is not common. However, people who have digestive or absorption problems, alcoholics, the elderly, and strict vegetarians are at risk of deficiency and can develop pernicious anemia.

Health Benefits

Vitamin B-12 is critical for maintaining a healthy nervous system, making DNA, protein synthesis, ensuring the production and health of red blood cells, and maintaining fertility. Your body reaps big benefits when you make sure you get enough of this critical nutrient.

- Supplementation with vitamin B-12, along with folic acid, can keep homocysteine levels down, which in turn can reduce your risk of atherosclerosis, heart attack, stroke, and other cardiovascular diseases.
- Insufficient levels of vitamin B-12 may result in an increase in DNA damage, which is a risk factor for cancer.
- Some research suggests that women who have low levels of vitamin B-12 are at greater risk of breast cancer.
- Several studies indicate that a low level of vitamin B-12 is a significant factor in dementia.
- Low levels of vitamin B-12 may play a role in depression, especially among older adults.
- Vitamin B-12 is necessary to help prevent or improve male infertility, as low levels can cause low sperm counts, abnormal sperm production, and reduced motility.

How Much Do I Need?

The DRI of vitamin B-12 for healthy adults is 2.4 mcg daily. Sublingual (under the tongue) tablets are recommended, as the nutrient is best absorbed by the body through the mucous membranes. Cyanocobalamin is the form usually found in supplements; the suggested dose is 100 to 400 mcg daily for anyone at risk for deficiency, and 500 to 1,000 mcg for those who are deficient. Signs and symptoms of a deficiency include pernicious anemia, mental confusion, elevated homocysteine levels, fatigue, depression, and memory loss.

Interactions

Vitamin B-12 supplements may interact with certain medications and other supplements.

- Use of metformin, phenytoin, primidone, and proton pump inhibitors (e.g., omeprazole [Prilosec], lansoprazole [Prevacid], esomeprazole [Nexium]) can reduce absorption of vitamin B-12.
- Large doses of folic acid can mask a vitamin B-12 deficiency.

• Potassium supplements can reduce absorption of vitamin B-12 in some people.

Food Sources

Food sources of vitamin B-12 include salmon, turkey, eggs, yogurt, nonfat milk, and cereals fortified with B-12.

VITAMIN C

Orange juice and vitamin C—these two just seem to go together naturally, and for good reason: oranges and orange juice are two of the most popular food sources of vitamin C. This water-soluble nutrient is essential to life, and needs to be replaced every day to help maintain health.

But if you thought that vitamin C's strong point was that it helped prevent the common cold and flu, recent studies show that just isn't so.

Health Benefits

A comprehensive review published in 2007 reported that, except for people who experience severe stress, taking daily supplements of vitamin C does very little to prevent colds or flu, or reduce their symptoms. However, vitamin C offers other important benefits, especially as an antioxidant, protecting the cells against free-radical damage. This function is vitally important, because cell damage from free radicals can cause cancer, cardiovascular disease, kidney and liver disease, lung disease, vision disorders, and many more medical problems.

Vitamin C also plays a key role in the development and maintenance of collagen (a component of bone, tendons, cartilage, teeth, and blood vessels), and it helps keep the gums and skin healthy. Your brain needs vitamin C so it can help manufacture norepinephrine, a chemical that affects mood. Vitamin C is also necessary for iron absorption, which is especially critical for menstruating women. Some evidence points to its ability to reduce cholesterol levels as well.

How Much Do I Need?

The DRI for vitamin C is 75 mg for women and 90 mg for men; women require 85 mg during pregnancy and 120 mg while breast-feeding. A typical range for supplementation is 500 to 1,000 mg daily.

Because it is possible to experience loose stool when taking higher levels of vitamin C, increase your dose gradually until you reach your goal, or a level you can tolerate without experiencing side effects. Supplements of vitamin C are usually available as ascorbic acid, which is best absorbed when it is combined with flavonoids.

Interactions

- Consider taking extra vitamin C if you are taking oral contraceptives or estrogen, because these hormones can reduce your body's supply of vitamin C.
- High levels of vitamin C (500 mg or greater) may increase the blood levels of aspirin and other nonsteroidal anti-inflammatory drugs, and/or acetaminophen.
- Vitamin C may reduce the absorption of propranolol, which is taken for high blood pressure.
- Vitamin C may increase the levels of tetracycline.

Food Sources

The best food sources of vitamin C are citrus (e.g., oranges, lemons, limes, grapefruit) as well as asparagus, bell peppers, blueberries, broccoli, brussels sprouts, cabbage, cantaloupe, cauliflower, kiwi, greens, papaya, parsley, strawberries, tomatoes, watermelon, and zucchini.

VITAMIN D

Vitamin D is known as the sunshine vitamin because, when the body is exposed to the ultraviolet rays from the sun, they trigger the synthesis of the vitamin in the skin. Vitamin D is also found in some foods.

Vitamin D exists in several forms, and each one has specific activities. Once vitamin D is in the body, it must be converted in the liver and kidneys into an active form of the vitamin, 1,25 dihydroxyvitamin D, which is actually a hormone. This hormone prompts the intestines to perform vital functions concerning bone health.

Health Benefits

Vitamin D is the driving force behind many critical functions in the body and also works along with other vitamins, minerals, and hormones. Here are a few of its tasks.

- Vitamin D increases the absorption of calcium and phosphorus in the intestines, which helps to form and maintain strong bones, and thus prevent osteoporosis and rickets.
- Results of a 2007 National Health Institutes–funded study found that women who took vitamin D and calcium had a sixty percent or greater reduction in cancer risk than women who did not take the vitamin.
- Higher levels of vitamin D in the blood have been linked with lower risk of colon and colorectal cancer.
- Low levels of vitamin D have been linked with atherosclerosis and congestive heart failure, based on several studies.
- Vitamin D can help relieve symptoms of asthma and, in pregnant women, a higher intake of the vitamin can decrease the risk of recurrent wheezing in infants and young children.

How Much Do I Need?

The current DRI is 200 IU per day (5 mg/day) for adults up to age 50, 400 IU per day from ages 51 to 70, and 600 IU daily thereafter. Vitamin D deficiency is most common among the elderly, as they often do not get adequate exposure to sunlight. People who live in high latitudes and anyone who has a disease characterized by fat malabsorption (e.g., Crohn's disease, celiac) may also be deficient.

Interactions

Vitamin D supplements may interact with medications and dietary supplements.

- If you are taking digoxin, talk to your doctor before taking vitamin D supplements because there is a risk of developing abnormal heart rhythms.
- Absorption of vitamin D is impaired if you use mineral oil.
- Use of Orlistat can reduce vitamin D levels in the body, so take this and other fat-soluble vitamin supplements at least two hours before or after taking Orlistat.
- Rifampin reduces vitamin D levels in the blood, so additional supplementation may be needed if you take this drug.

Food Sources

Foods that contain vitamin D include eggs (yolk), nonfat milk, salmon, and tuna. Also look for foods that have been fortified with vitamin D, including breakfast cereals and dairy products.

VITAMIN E

Vitamin E is not one but actually a group of eight different compounds: four in the tocopherol family and four in the tocotrienol family, with alpha, beta, gamma, and delta varieties in each family. Of the eight, alpha-tocopherol is the most common form of vitamin E.

The term "tocopherol" means "to bring forth children," which refers to the fact that when vitamin E was first identified, its absence was found to make lab rats infertile. We now know that vitamin E has many other qualities as well.

Health Benefits

Vitamin E is a powerful antioxidant that protects against free-radical damage, especially in the nervous system, muscles, eyes, and blood cells. Yet a confusing and disturbing study released in November 2004 reported that vitamin E supplements were linked with a slightly increased risk of death. However, many experts later questioned those results given that most of the patients in the studies were elderly and had cancer, heart disease, or other chronic illnesses, and were already at increased risk of dying.

- Several large studies have found that vitamin E supplements can reduce the risk of heart disease by about forty percent. It does this by reducing the activity of bad cholesterol and the formation of plaque in the arteries, which in turn helps prevent the development of blood clots.
- A few studies of vitamin E suggest it can reduce the risk of cataracts and macular degeneration.
- Vitamin E may also ease symptoms of rheumatoid arthritis.
- Symptoms of PMS and fibrocystic breast syndrome may also be reduced if you take vitamin E; 400 IU daily is suggested.
- Supplementation with vitamin E may boost immunity and help protect against the common cold and flu.
- Some studies suggest vitamin E may reduce the risk of prostate, breast, and bladder cancer. In the Alpha-tocopherol, Beta-carotene Cancer Prevention Study, for example, alpha-tocopherol (50 mg daily) reduced prostate cancer incidence by 32 percent.

How Much Do I Need?

The DRI for vitamin E for adults is 22 to 33 IU daily, which translates into 15 to 22 mg. Yet most Americans get only fifty to seventy-five percent of that amount. Because tocopherols and tocotrienols have different effects on the body, some experts suggest taking a supplement that contains both mixed tocopherols and mixed tocotrienols. Andrew Weil, MD, recommends taking at least 80 mg of these mixtures daily; an alternative is 400 IU daily of mixed natural tocopherols.

Interactions

Interactions between vitamin E and a few medications and supplements have been noted.

- Use of anticonvulsant or cholesterol-lowering drugs can significantly reduce the body's supply of vitamin E.
- Prolonged use of mineral oil can reduce the body's supply of vitamin E.
- Vitamin E is very dependent on vitamin C, vitamin B-3, selenium, and glutathione, which means a diet high in vitamin E cannot be optimally effective unless it is also rich in foods that provide these other nutrients.
- High doses of vitamin E (1,000 mg or more) can interfere with vitamin K in the body.

Food Sources

Good to excellent food sources of vitamin E include almonds, broccoli, greens, kiwi, mango, sunflower seed kernels and oil, and wheat germ oil.

ZINC

Nearly every cell in the body contains zinc, a mineral that is a cofactor for (stimulates the activity of) more than a hundred enzymes, especially those necessary for metabolizing protein, carbohydrates, fats, and alcohol. More than fifty percent of the body's supply of zinc is found in the muscles; the rest is distributed mainly in the skin, eyes, bones, prostate, testes, and kidneys.

Health Benefits

Zinc plays a significant role in many processes, including protein synthesis, tissue growth, wound healing, blood clotting, bone development, sperm production, and thyroid function. It is also important in the prevention and treatment of various medical conditions.

- Zinc is important in promoting the immune system, and there is evidence that it can reduce the symptoms of the common cold and fight infections.
- In its role as an antioxidant, zinc helps protect the macula in the eye, which means it has a role in preventing macular degeneration.
- Infertile men typically have low levels of zinc, and studies indicate that supplementing with zinc (15 mg twice daily) can benefit sperm production and the male reproductive system.

How Much Do I Need?

The DRIs for zinc are 8 mg for women and 11 mg for men. Zinc is best absorbed by the body when it is taken with food that contains protein. When choosing a zinc supplement, look for forms that are more easily absorbed, including zinc picolinate, zinc citrate, zinc acetate, and zinc glycerate. The least easily absorbed is zinc sulfate, a form that can also cause stomach distress. Zinc lozenges, which are often used to prevent and treat the common cold, can cause nausea, mouth irritation, stomach pain, and a bad taste in the mouth.

Taking too much zinc (40 mg or greater) can impair the absorption of iron and copper, so be sure you note the amount of zinc in any supplements you are taking. Zinc deficiency is not common except among alcoholics; it is also seen in people who have digestive disorders or who have chronic diarrhea, and in people who are malnourished.

Interactions

Zinc supplements react with a few other substances. Here's what we know so far:

- Zinc may decrease the amount of oral quinolones (e.g., ciprofloxacin, levofloxacin, norfloxacin, ofloxacin) and nonsteroidal anti-inflammatory drugs (e.g., ibuprofen, naproxen, aspirin) your body absorbs, and thus impact the effectiveness of these drugs.

- Do not take zinc supplements at the same time you take copper, iron, or phosphorus. To ensure you get the benefits from all these nutrients, take zinc about two hours before or after taking the other supplements.

Food Sources

Although oysters are often touted as the best source of zinc, many other foods provide a good amount, including almonds, beans (dried), fortified cereals, nonfat milk, oatmeal, peas, pumpkin seeds, walnuts, and yogurt.

GLOSSARY

ANTHOCYANINS: Plant pigments that are responsible for the red, blue, and purple fruits, vegetables, flowers, and cereal grains. Anthocyanins are antioxidants, and are believed to be useful in the treatment of vision and circulatory problems.

ANTIOXIDANTS: Compounds that prevent damage to cells from oxidation or from molecules known as free radicals. The body can make its own antioxidants but relies heavily on antioxidants from the diet. Dietary antioxidants include vitamins C and E, beta-carotene, selenium, copper, zinc, and phytonutrients

BETA-CAROTENE: A type of carotenoid and a plant pigment that is converted into vitamin A in the body. It is also known as provitamin A.

BIOFLAVONOIDS: Compounds found in fruits that contain vitamin C. They are sometimes included in vitamin C supplements.

CAROTENOIDS: Fat-soluble plant pigments that the body converts into vitamin A.

COENZYME: A nonprotein molecule that binds with a protein molecule in order to form an active enzyme, which can then participate in chemical processes.

DAILY VALUE: A term that replaces the RDA (Recommended Dietary Allowance) on food labels. It refers to the percentage of the recommended daily amount of a substance that each serving or dose provides.

DIETARY REFERENCE INTAKES (DRIS): A set of values that are the standards for nutrient intake for healthy people. The values are based on the average requirements for males and females of all ages and include Estimated Average Requirements (EAR), Recommended Dietary Allowances (RDA), Tolerable Upper Intake Levels (UL), and Adequate Intake (AI) values.

DIHYDROTESTOSTERONE: A metabolite of the male hormone testosterone. It is three times more potent than testosterone, and is often associated with male baldness and prostate problems.

DOCOSAHEXAENOIC ACID (DHA): A type of omega-3 essential fatty acid found in fatty fish, such as salmon, tuna, and herring.

EICOSAPENTAENOIC ACID (EPA): A type of omega-3 essential fatty acid. The body has a limited ability to make EPA by converting alpha-linolenic acid (ALA).

ESSENTIAL FATTY ACIDS: The two fatty acids—linoleic and alpha-linolenic (ALA)—that the body requires but cannot manufacture, which means they must be obtained through diet and/or supplements.

FAT-SOLUBLE VITAMINS: Vitamins that can be dissolved in fat and are stored in fat tissue. They include vitamins A, D, E, and K.

FLAVONOIDS: Any of a large group of phytonutrients that are plant pigments; also called bioflavonoids.

FREE RADICALS: Unstable molecules that attach themselves to other molecules and damage cells in the process.

HOMOCYSTEINE: An amino acid produced by the body from another amino acid (methionine), and then converted into other amino acids. High levels of homocysteine are associated with an increased risk of cardiovascular disease.

LIGNAN: A member of a group of substances found in plants that have demonstrated anticancer and estrogenic properties.

NEUROTRANSMITTERS: Chemicals produced by the brain and nerves that transmit and change nerve messages and make it possible for people to feel and think.

NOREPINEPHRINE: A chemical produced by some nerve cells and in the adrenal gland. It can perform as a hormone and as a neurotransmitter.

OSTEOBLASTS: Cells that make the framework of new bone.

OSTEOCALCIN: A type of protein found in bone. It is secreted by osteoblasts—cells that help make bone.

OSTEOCLASTS: Cells that break down bone.

PHYTOESTROGENS: These plant chemicals are similar in structure to the hormone estrogen, but have a significantly reduced estrogen effect. Two main types of phytoestrogens are lignans and isoflavones.

PHYTONUTRIENTS: A substance derived from plants ("phyto"), especially one that is neither a vitamin nor mineral, that is beneficial to health.

POLYPHENOLS: A type of phytonutrient and potent antioxidants. The word literally means "many phenols," and a phenol is a type of carbon-based molecule.

PHYTOSTEROLS: Plant-based compounds (also called plant sterols) that can compete with dietary cholesterol and be absorbed by the intestines, which means phytosterols can lower cholesterol levels.

RESVERATROL: A type of polyphenol and a potent antioxidant that is credited with inhibiting the growth of certain cancer cells and of reducing inflammation.

WATER-SOLUBLE VITAMINS: Vitamins that the body does not store, so they need to be replaced daily. Examples include the B vitamins and vitamin C.

GENERAL HEALTH, NUTRITION, AND SUPPLEMENT RESOURCES

Center for Food Safety and Applied Nutrition
http://www.cfsan.fda.gov/~dms/supplmnt.html

Information on dietary supplements.

Consumer Lab
www.consumerlab.com

Provides independent test results on nutrition products.

Dietary Supplement Information Bureau
http://www.supplementinfo.org/

Provides information on the responsible use of vitamins, minerals, herbs, and specialty supplements. Funded by scientific, industry, and education groups.

Dietary Supplements Labels Database
http://dietarysupplements.nlm.nih.gov/dietary/

Provides information about the ingredients in more than 2,000 selected brands of dietary supplements. Allows you to compare ingredients in different brands without leaving the house.

Food and Nutrition Information Center
http://fnic.nal.usda.gov/nal_display/index.php?info_center=4&tax_level=1&tax_subject=274

Information on dietary supplements.

Health A to Z
www.healthatoz.com

Comprehensive information on consumer health topics.

Health Central
www.healthcentral.com

Comprehensive information on consumer health topics.

Linus Pauling Institute
http://lpi.oregonstate.edu/infocenter/

Micronutrient research for optimum health.

Mayo Clinic
www.mayoclinic.com

Comprehensive overviews on a wide range of consumer health topics.

National Agricultural Library, USDA
http://www.nutrition.gov/nal_display/index.php?info_center=11&tax_level=1&tax_subject=382

Information on food and human nutrition.

National Center for Complementary and Alternative Medicine

http://nccam.nih.gov/health/supplements.htm

Governmental site on complementary and alternative nutrition and medicine.

National Institutes of Health

http://health.nih.gov

Provides information on consumer health topics, clinical trials, research, and more.

Nutritional Tree

http://www.nutritionaltree.com/default.aspx

Publishes consumers' reviews of nutritional products; does not accept any advertising.

US Pharmacopeia

www.usp.org

An independent public health organization; offers information on dietary supplements.

Wrong Diagnosis

www.wrongdiagnosis.com

Provides information on symptoms, diagnosis, and misdiagnosis of more than 10,000 medical conditions.